SHORT-COURSE CHEMOTHERAPY FOR TUBERCULOSIS

The transcript of a Witness Seminar held by the Wellcome Trust Centre for the History of Medicine at UCL, London, on 3 February 2004

Edited by D A Christie and E M Tansey

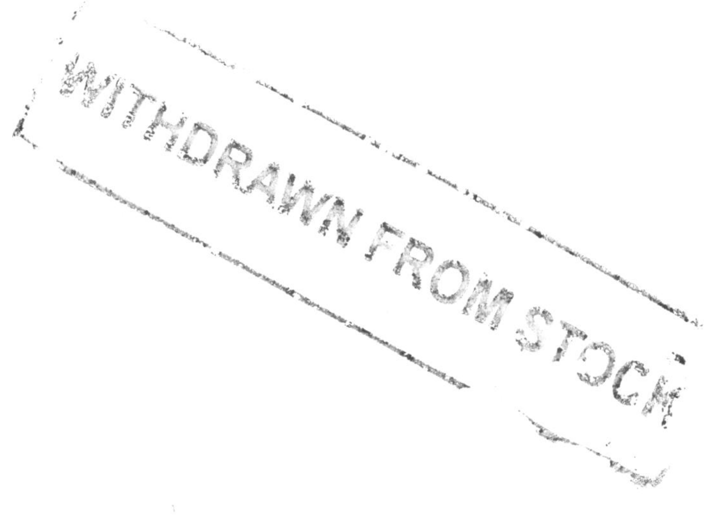

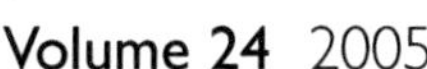

Volume 24 2005

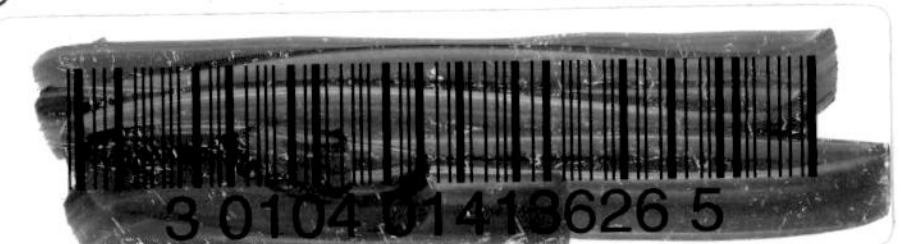

First published by the Wellcome Trust Centre
for the History of Medicine at UCL, 2005

The Wellcome Trust Centre for the History of Medicine
at University College London is funded by the Wellcome Trust,
which is a registered charity, no. 210183.

ISBN 0 85484 104 0

Histmed logo images courtesy of the Wellcome Library, London.

Design and production: Julie Wood at Shift Key Design 020 7241 3704

All volumes freely available online following the links to publications at www.ucl.ac.uk/histmed

Technology Transfer in Britain: The case of monoclonal antibodies; Self and Non-Self: A history of autoimmunity; Endogenous Opiates; The Committee on Safety of Drugs • Making the Human Body Transparent: The impact of NMR and MRI; Research in General Practice; Drugs in Psychiatric Practice; The MRC Common Cold Unit • Early Heart Transplant Surgery in the UK • Haemophilia: Recent history of clinical management • Looking at the Unborn: Historical aspects of obstetric ultrasound • Post Penicillin Antibiotics: From acceptance to resistance? • Clinical Research in Britain, 1950–1980 • Intestinal Absorption • Origins of Neonatal Intensive Care in the UK • British Contributions to Medical Research and Education in Africa after the Second World War • Childhood Asthma and Beyond • Maternal Care • Population-based Research in South Wales: The MRC Pneumoconiosis Research Unit and the MRC Epidemiology Unit • Peptic Ulcer: Rise and fall • Leukaemia • The MRC Applied Psychology Unit • Genetic Testing • Foot and Mouth Disease: The 1967 outbreak and its aftermath • Environmental Toxicology: The legacy of *Silent Spring* • Cystic Fibrosis • Innovation in Pain Management • The Rhesus Factor and Disease Prevention

CONTENTS

ILLUSTRATIONS AND CREDITS

WITNESS SEMINARS: MEETINGS AND PUBLICATIONS[1]

In 1990 the Wellcome Trust created a History of Twentieth Century Medicine Group, as part of the Academic Unit of the Wellcome Institute for the History of Medicine, to bring together clinicians, scientists, historians and others interested in contemporary medical history. Among a number of other initiatives the format of Witness Seminars, used by the Institute of Contemporary British History to address issues of recent political history, was adopted, to promote interaction between these different groups, to emphasize the potential benefits of working jointly, and to encourage the creation and deposit of archival sources for present and future use. In June 1999 the Governors of the Wellcome Trust decided that it would be appropriate for the Academic Unit to enjoy a more formal academic affiliation and turned the Unit into the Wellcome Trust Centre for the History of Medicine at University College London from 1 October 2000. The Wellcome Trust continues to fund the Witness Seminar programme via its support for the Wellcome Trust Centre.

The Witness Seminar is a particularly specialized form of oral history, where several people associated with a particular set of circumstances or events are invited to come together to discuss, debate, and agree or disagree about their memories. To date, the History of Twentieth Century Medicine Group has held 40 such meetings, most of which have been published, as listed on pages xi–xviii.

Subjects are usually proposed by, or through, members of the Programme Committee of the Group, and once an appropriate topic has been agreed, suitable participants are identified and invited. This inevitably leads to further contacts, and more suggestions of people to invite. As the organization of the meeting progresses, a flexible outline plan for the meeting is devised, usually with assistance from the meeting's chairman, and some participants are invited to 'set the ball rolling' on particular themes, by speaking for a short period to initiate and stimulate further discussion.

Each meeting is fully recorded, the tapes are transcribed and the unedited transcript is immediately sent to every participant. Each is asked to check his

---

[1] The following text also appears in the 'Introduction' to recent volumes of *Wellcome Witnesses to Twentieth Century Medicine* published by the Wellcome Trust and the Wellcome Trust Centre for the History of Medicine at University College London.

or her own contributions and to provide brief biographical details. The editors turn the transcript into readable text, and participants' minor corrections and comments are incorporated into that text, while biographical and bibliographical details are added as footnotes, as are more substantial comments and additional material provided by participants. The final scripts are then sent to every contributor, accompanied by forms assigning copyright to the Wellcome Trust. Copies of all additional correspondence received during the editorial process are deposited with the records of each meeting in Archives and Manuscripts, Wellcome Library, London.

As with all our meetings, we hope that even if the precise details of some of the technical sections are not clear to the non-specialist, the sense and significance of the events will be understandable. Our aim is for the volumes that emerge from these meetings to inform those with a general interest in the history of modern medicine and medical science; to provide historians with new insights, fresh material for study, and further themes for research; and to emphasize to the participants that events of the recent past, of their own working lives, are of proper and necessary concern to historians.

ACKNOWLEDGEMENTS

Short-course chemotherapy for tuberculosis was suggested as a suitable topic for a Witness Seminar by Dr Owen McCarthy. He provided many of the names of individuals to be invited, and helped decide on the topics to be discussed. We thank him for his input. We are particularly grateful to Professor Linda Bryder for writing the Introduction to these published proceedings and to Dr David Girling for his excellent chairing of the occasion and for his help with the planning of the meeting. Dr Lise Wilkinson kindly read the edited transcript for general sense and understandability. We thank Dr Joseph Angel, Sir John Crofton, Dr David Girling and Professor Denny Mitchison for additional help with the text. Mrs Gaye Fox and Dr Joseph Angel kindly provided the illustrations.

As with all our meetings, we depend a great deal on our colleagues at the Wellcome Trust to ensure their smooth running: the Audiovisual Department, the Medical Photographic Library and Mrs Tracy Tillotson of the Wellcome Library; Ms Julie Wood, who has supervised the design and production of this volume; our indexer, Ms Liza Furnival, and our readers, Ms Lucy Moore and Mr Simon Reynolds. Mrs Jaqui Carter is our transcriber, and Mrs Wendy Kutner and Mrs Lois Reynolds assist us in running the meetings. Finally we thank the Wellcome Trust for supporting this programme.

Tilli Tansey

Daphne Christie

Wellcome Trust Centre for the History of Medicine at UCL

HISTORY OF TWENTIETH CENTURY MEDICINE WITNESS SEMINARS, 1993–2005

1993 **Monoclonal antibodies**
Organizers: Dr E M Tansey and Dr Peter Catterall

1994 **The early history of renal transplantation**
Organizer: Dr Stephen Lock

Pneumoconiosis of coal workers
Organizer: Dr E M Tansey

1995 **Self and non-self: A history of autoimmunity**
Organizers: Sir Christopher Booth and Dr E M Tansey

Ashes to ashes: The history of smoking and health
Organizers: Dr Stephen Lock and Dr E M Tansey

Oral contraceptives
Organizers: Dr Lara Marks and Dr E M Tansey

Endogenous opiates
Organizer: Dr E M Tansey

1996 **Committee on Safety of Drugs**
Organizers: Dr Stephen Lock and Dr E M Tansey

Making the body more transparent: The impact of nuclear magnetic resonance and magnetic resonance imaging
Organizer: Sir Christopher Booth

1997 **Research in general practice**
Organizers: Dr Ian Tait and Dr E M Tansey

Drugs in psychiatric practice
Organizers: Dr David Healy and Dr E M Tansey

The MRC Common Cold Unit
Organizers: Dr David Tyrrell and Dr E M Tansey

The first heart transplant in the UK
Organizer: Professor Tom Treasure

1998	**Haemophilia: Recent history of clinical management** Organizers: Professor Christine Lee and Dr E M Tansey
	Obstetric ultrasound: Historical perspectives Organizers: Dr Malcolm Nicolson, Mr John Fleming and Dr E M Tansey
	Post penicillin antibiotics Organizers: Dr Robert Bud and Dr E M Tansey
	Clinical research in Britain, 1950–1980 Organizers: Dr David Gordon and Dr E M Tansey
1999	**Intestinal absorption** Organizers: Sir Christopher Booth and Dr E M Tansey
	The MRC Epidemiology Unit (South Wales) Organizers: Dr Andy Ness and Dr E M Tansey
	Neonatal intensive care Organizers: Professor Osmund Reynolds and Dr E M Tansey
	British contributions to medicine in Africa after the Second World War Organizers: Dr Mary Dobson, Dr Maureen Malowany, Dr Gordon Cook and Dr E M Tansey
2000	**Childhood asthma, and beyond** Organizers: Dr Chris O'Callaghan and Dr Daphne Christie
	Peptic ulcer: Rise and fall Organizers: Sir Christopher Booth, Professor Roy Pounder and Dr E M Tansey
	Maternal care Organizers: Dr Irvine Loudon and Dr Daphne Christie
2001	**Leukaemia** Organizers: Professor Sir David Weatherall, Professor John Goldman, Sir Christopher Booth and Dr Daphne Christie
	The MRC Applied Psychology Unit Organizers: Dr Geoff Bunn and Dr Daphne Christie
	Genetic testing Organizers: Professor Doris Zallen and Dr Daphne Christie

Foot and mouth disease: the 1967 outbreak and its aftermath
Organizers: Dr Abigail Woods, Dr Daphne Christie and Dr David Aickin

2002 **Environmental toxicology: The legacy of *Silent Spring***
Organizers: Dr Robert Flanagan and Dr Daphne Christie

Cystic fibrosis
Organizers: Dr James Littlewood and Dr Daphne Christie

Innovation in pain management
Organizers: Professor David Clark and Dr Daphne Christie

2003 **Thrombolysis**
Organizers: Mr Robert Arnott and Dr Daphne Christie

Beyond the asylum: Anti-psychiatry and care in the community
Organizers: Dr Mark Jackson and Dr Daphne Christie

The Rhesus factor and disease prevention
Organizers: Professor Doris Zallen and Dr Daphne Christie

Platelets in thrombosis and other disorders
Organizers: Professor Gustav Born and Dr Daphne Christie

2004 **Short-course chemotherapy for tuberculosis**
Organizers: Dr Owen McCarthy and Dr Daphne Christie

Prenatal corticosteroids for reducing morbidity and mortality associated with preterm birth
Organizers: Sir Iain Chalmers and Dr Daphne Christie

Public health in the 1980s and 1990s: Decline and rise?
Organizers: Professor Virginia Berridge, Dr Niki Ellis and Dr Daphne Christie

2005 **The history of cholesterol, atherosclerosis and coronary disease**
Organizers: Professor Michael Oliver and Dr Daphne Christie

Development of physics applied to medicine in the UK, 1945–90
Organizers: Professor John Clifton and Dr Daphne Christie

PUBLISHED MEETINGS

"...Few books are so intellectually stimulating or uplifting".
Journal of the Royal Society of Medicine (1999) **92:** 206–8,
review of vols 1 and 2

"...This is oral history at its best...all the volumes make compulsive reading...they are, primarily, important historical records".
British Medical Journal (2002) **325**: 1119, review of the series

Technology transfer in Britain: The case of monoclonal antibodies
Self and non-self: A history of autoimmunity
Endogenous opiates
The Committee on Safety of Drugs
In: Tansey E M, Catterall P P, Christie D A, Willhoft S V, Reynolds L A. (eds) (1997) *Wellcome Witnesses to Twentieth Century Medicine.* Volume 1. London: The Wellcome Trust, 135pp. ISBN 1 869835 79 4

Making the human body transparent: The impact of NMR and MRI
Research in general practice
Drugs in psychiatric practice
The MRC Common Cold Unit
In: Tansey E M, Christie D A, Reynolds L A. (eds) (1998) *Wellcome Witnesses to Twentieth Century Medicine.* Volume 2. London: The Wellcome Trust, 282pp. ISBN 1 869835 39 5

Early heart transplant surgery in the UK
In: Tansey E M, Reynolds L A. (eds) (1999) *Wellcome Witnesses to Twentieth Century Medicine.* Volume 3. London: The Wellcome Trust, 72pp. ISBN 1 841290 07 6

Haemophilia: Recent history of clinical management
In: Tansey E M, Christie D A. (eds) (1999) *Wellcome Witnesses to Twentieth Century Medicine.* Volume 4. London: The Wellcome Trust, 90pp. ISBN 1 841290 08 4

Looking at the unborn: Historical aspects of obstetric ultrasound
In: Tansey E M, Christie D A. (eds) (2000) *Wellcome Witnesses to Twentieth*

Century Medicine. Volume 5. London: The Wellcome Trust, 80pp.
ISBN 1 841290 11 4

Post penicillin antibiotics: From acceptance to resistance?
In: Tansey E M, Reynolds L A. (eds) (2000) *Wellcome Witnesses to Twentieth Century Medicine*. Volume 6. London: The Wellcome Trust, 71pp.
ISBN 1 841290 12 2

Clinical research in Britain, 1950–1980
In: Reynolds L A, Tansey E M. (eds) (2000) *Wellcome Witnesses to Twentieth Century Medicine*. Volume 7. London: The Wellcome Trust, 74pp.
ISBN 1 841290 16 5

Intestinal absorption
In: Christie D A, Tansey E M. (eds) (2000) *Wellcome Witnesses to Twentieth Century Medicine*. Volume 8. London: The Wellcome Trust, 81pp.
ISBN 1 841290 17 3

Neonatal intensive care
In: Christie D A, Tansey E M. (eds) (2001) *Wellcome Witnesses to Twentieth Century Medicine*. Volume 9. London: The Wellcome Trust Centre for the History of Medicine at UCL, 84pp. ISBN 0 854840 76 1

British contributions to medical research and education in Africa after the Second World War
In: Reynolds L A, Tansey E M. (eds) (2001) *Wellcome Witnesses to Twentieth Century Medicine*. Volume 10. London: The Wellcome Trust Centre for the History of Medicine at UCL, 93pp. ISBN 0 854840 77 X

Childhood asthma and beyond
In: Reynolds L A, Tansey E M. (eds) (2001) *Wellcome Witnesses to Twentieth Century Medicine*. Volume 11. London: The Wellcome Trust Centre for the History of Medicine at UCL, 74pp. ISBN 0 854840 78 8

Maternal care
In: Christie D A, Tansey E M. (eds) (2001) *Wellcome Witnesses to Twentieth Century Medicine*. Volume 12. London: The Wellcome Trust Centre for the History of Medicine at UCL, 88pp. ISBN 0 854840 79 6

Population-based research in south Wales: The MRC Pneumoconiosis Research Unit and the MRC Epidemiology Unit
In: Ness A R, Reynolds L A, Tansey E M. (eds) (2002) *Wellcome Witnesses to Twentieth Century Medicine*. Volume 13. London: The Wellcome Trust Centre for the History of Medicine at UCL, 74pp. ISBN 0 854840 81 8

Peptic ulcer: Rise and fall
In: Christie D A, Tansey E M. (eds) (2002) *Wellcome Witnesses to Twentieth Century Medicine*. Volume 14. London: The Wellcome Trust Centre for the History of Medicine at UCL, 143pp. ISBN 0 854840 84 2

Leukaemia
In: Christie D A, Tansey E M. (eds) (2003) *Wellcome Witnesses to Twentieth Century Medicine*. Volume 15. London: The Wellcome Trust Centre for the History of Medicine at UCL, 86pp. ISBN 0 85484 087 7

The MRC Applied Psychology Unit
In: Reynolds L A, Tansey E M. (eds) (2003) *Wellcome Witnesses to Twentieth Century Medicine*. Volume 16. London: The Wellcome Trust Centre for the History of Medicine at UCL, 94pp. ISBN 0 85484 088 5

Genetic testing
In: Christie D A, Tansey E M. (eds) (2003) *Wellcome Witnesses to Twentieth Century Medicine*. Volume 17. London: The Wellcome Trust Centre for the History of Medicine at UCL, 130pp. ISBN 0 85484 094 X

Foot and mouth disease: The 1967 outbreak and its aftermath
In: Reynolds L A, Tansey E M. (eds) (2003) *Wellcome Witnesses to Twentieth Century Medicine*. Volume 18. London: The Wellcome Trust Centre for the History of Medicine at UCL, 114pp. ISBN 0 85484 096 6

Environmental toxicology: The legacy of *Silent Spring*
In: Christie D A, Tansey E M. (eds) (2004) *Wellcome Witnesses to Twentieth Century Medicine*. Volume 19. London: The Wellcome Trust Centre for the History of Medicine at UCL, 132pp. ISBN 0 85484 091 5

Cystic fibrosis
In: Christie D A, Tansey E M. (eds) (2004) *Wellcome Witnesses to Twentieth Century Medicine*. Volume 20. London: The Wellcome Trust Centre for the History of Medicine at UCL, 120pp. ISBN 0 85484 086 9

Innovation in pain management
In: Reynolds L A, Tansey E M. (eds) (2004) *Wellcome Witnesses to Twentieth Century Medicine.* Volume 21. London: The Wellcome Trust Centre for the History of Medicine at UCL, 125pp. ISBN 0 85484 097 4

The Rhesus factor and disease prevention
In: Zallen D T, Christie D A, Tansey E M. (eds) (2004) *Wellcome Witnesses to Twentieth Century Medicine.* Volume 22. London: The Wellcome Trust Centre for the History of Medicine at UCL, 98pp. ISBN 0 85484 099 0

The recent history of platelets in thrombosis and other disorders
In: Reynolds L A, Tansey E M. (eds) (2005) *Wellcome Witnesses to Twentieth Century Medicine.* Volume 23. London: The Wellcome Trust Centre for the History of Medicine at UCL, 186pp. ISBN 0 85484 103 2

Short-course chemotherapy for tuberculosis
In: Christie D A, Tansey E M. (eds) (2005) *Wellcome Witnesses to Twentieth Century Medicine.* Volume 24. London: The Wellcome Trust Centre for the History of Medicine at UCL, this volume. ISBN 0 85484 104 0

Prenatal corticosteroids for reducing morbidity and mortality associated with preterm birth
In: Reynolds L A, Tansey E M. (eds) (2005) *Wellcome Witnesses to Twentieth Century Medicine.* Volume 25. London: The Wellcome Trust Centre for the History of Medicine at UCL. In press.

Public health in the 1980s and 1990s: Decline and rise?
In: Berridge V, Christie D A, Tansey E M. (eds) (2005) *Wellcome Witnesses to Twentieth Century Medicine.* Volume 26. London: The Wellcome Trust Centre for the History of Medicine at UCL. In press.

Volumes 1–12 cost £5 plus postage, with volumes 13–20 at £10 each. Orders of four or more volumes receive a 20 per cent discount. All 20 published volumes in the series are available at the special price of £115 plus postage. To order a copy contact t.tillotson@wellcome.ac.uk or by phone: +44 (0)20 7611 8486; or fax: +44 (0)20 7611 8703.

All volumes are freely available online under publications at www.ucl.ac.uk/histmed A hard copy of volumes 21–24 can be ordered from www.amazon.co.uk; www.amazon.com; and all good booksellers.

Other publications

Technology transfer in Britain: The case of monoclonal antibodies
In: Tansey E M, Catterall P P. (1993) *Contemporary Record* 9: 409–44.

Monoclonal antibodies: A witness seminar on contemporary medical history
In: Tansey E M, Catterall P P. (1994) *Medical History* 38: 322–7.

Chronic pulmonary disease in South Wales coalmines: An eye-witness account of the MRC surveys (1937–42)
In: P D'Arcy Hart, edited and annotated by E M Tansey. (1998) *Social History of Medicine* 11: 459–68.

Ashes to Ashes – The history of smoking and health
In: Lock S P, Reynolds L A, Tansey E M. (eds) (1998) Amsterdam: Rodopi BV, 228pp. ISBN 90420 0396 0 (Hfl 125) (hardback). Reprinted 2003.

Witnessing medical history. An interview with Dr Rosemary Biggs
Professor Christine Lee and Dr Charles Rizza (interviewers). (1998) *Haemophilia* 4: 769–77.

Witnessing the Witnesses: Pitfalls and potentials of the Witness Seminar in twentieth century medicine
By E M Tansey. In: Doel R, Soderqvist T. (eds) (2005) *Writing Recent Science: The historiography of contemporary science, technology and medicine.* London: Routledge.

INTRODUCTION

When Archie Cochrane, the British medical researcher who contributed so much to the development of epidemiology as a science, judged which speciality in medicine deserved the gold medal for being the most evidence-based, he gave a 'Bradford' (a 'gold medal' named after epidemiologist Sir Austin Bradford Hill) to tuberculosis specialists, and he gave obstetrics the wooden spoon (page 65).[1] This witness seminar supports that assessment of tuberculosis, providing a fascinating account of laboratory research, clinical trials, and treatment regimens since the MRC randomized controlled trials on the first antituberculosis drug, streptomycin, led by Bradford Hill, Philip D'Arcy Hart and Marc Daniels in 1948.[2]

Standard treatment for pulmonary tuberculosis in the 1960s consisted of administering streptomycin for three months, and the drugs isoniazid and PAS (para-aminosalicylic acid) for 18 months to two years. This seemed to work. Dr Kenneth Citron from the Royal Brompton Hospital, London, who had been consultant adviser on tuberculosis to the Department of Health, tells us of a follow-up study in England in 1971 showing that 90 per cent of patients were treated for the allocated time and that all but 2 per cent became culture-negative, and on a follow-up for three to seven years none had relapsed (page 67). The drive for a shorter course of treatment came not from Britain, with its well-staffed tuberculosis clinics and army of tuberculosis health visitors, but from developing countries with their under-developed health services, where tuberculosis was rife and which later also had to contend with the HIV/AIDS epidemic. The two-year course of treatment was not only expensive but there was also a major problem of patient compliance and supervision. As a result of various trials, primarily carried out in India and East Africa, by the end of the 1970s the accepted course of treatment had become an eight-month regimen, consisting of two months of streptomycin/isoniazid/rifampicin/pyrazinamide, followed by six months of thiacetazone and isoniazid. This was subsequently reduced to six months, a change embraced wholeheartedly by health workers in these countries, and endorsed by the International Union against Tuberculosis and Lung Disease and the World Health Organization.

---

[1] Cochrane (1979): 1–11.

[2] Medical Research Council (1948); For details of Bradford Hill's first attempt to introduce the concept of randomization in controlled trials, see Wilkinson (1997). See also D'Arcy Hart (1999); Chalmers (2005): 309–34.

Speakers at the seminar highlighted the important trials which led to the changes – Professor Wallace Fox's famous 1959 trial in Madras on sanatorium versus home treatment, which contributed to the trend of closing of tuberculosis sanatoria by the end of the 1960s (page 32).[3] The East African study, known affectionately as 'Study R', was the first short-course chemotherapy study, carried out in 42 centres in East Africa and Zambia, and coordinated by Dr Amina Jindani, one of the seminar's witnesses. This study along with one in Hong Kong, brought together the three drugs, isoniazid – rifampicin and pyrazinamide – for the first time.

Dr David Girling, who was involved with the International Union Against Tuberculosis and Lung Disease, listed the impressive geographical spread of trials, including East and Central Africa, Hong Kong, Singapore, Transkei, Poland, East Germany, Czechoslovakia, Algeria, Finland, Argentina and Korea, as well as the UK and France. He commented, 'I think this is probably one of the largest international combined research enterprises that has been conducted in the history of medicine' (page 26), and Ian Campbell noted significantly that it was not driven by pharmaceutical companies.

For the historian of medicine, the insights into the use of streptomycin are of particular interest. Streptomycin is always given pride of place in medical history books as the subject of the first randomized clinical trial. At the seminar it was pointed out that it was not, as commonly believed, the very first 'properly controlled multicentre trial'; that honour goes to the 1944 antibiotic patulin trial, organized by Philip D'Arcy Hart, who also ran the streptomycin trial (page 35).[4] The absence of D'Arcy Hart at the witness seminar was regretted, although it was pointed out that his 104th birthday was imminent!

The streptomycin trial was considered by participants to be important for another reason. Sir John Crofton, Professor of Respiratory Diseases and Tuberculosis at the University of Edinburgh from 1952 to 1977, explained that it was the first important new antibiotic after penicillin. Patients on penicillin did not develop resistance under treatment; patients on streptomycin did. In Crofton's view, this was a grim new phenomenon and a

---

[3] Tuberculosis Chemotherapy Centre, Madras (1959).

[4] Medical Research Council, Patulin Clinical Trials Committee (1944); Clinical trials ran from December 1943 to April 1944, supervised by Dr Joan Faulkner. See also D'Arcy Hart (1999); Chalmers and Clarke (2004); The James Lind Library (www.jameslindlibrary.org) visited 7 June 2005.

forewarning of things to come. He also commented on the rather negative initial response to this famous trial, until other drugs came along. Professor Denis Mitchison, Professor of Bacteriology at the Royal Postgraduate Medical School at Hammersmith Hospital, also thought streptomycin was 'not a very good drug'. Professor Peter Ormerod, another former consultant adviser on tuberculosis to the Department of Health, provided a more personal touch. He recalled as a seven-year-old experiencing intramuscular streptomycin: 'As someone who had very little buttock at the age of seven, it was not a very pleasant experience' – he had to sleep on his front for three months! (Page 31.) Some 'streptomycin defenders', we are told, kept it for 'fractious patients', who received injections to ensure compliance (page 39).

One of the advantages of a witness seminar, not normally captured in the written record, is the sense of 'being there' when important research is being carried out. Thus you have Dr Joseph Angel's reference to research worker Tony Jenkins 'drowning in sputum' (page 72), and Dr Jindani's encounters with giraffes and elephants in Africa (page 21). Professor Janet Darbyshire, who coordinated MRC clinical trials in Africa, also described encounters with elephants and lions, and spending hours and hours in Land Rovers (page 18). Moreover, the way in which research was conducted in 1950s is often forgotten in our computer age. Mrs Gaye Fox described research conditions in Madras in the 1950s – 'no air conditioning at all for the first two years, no machines for sorting out statistical cards, hence the cards were sorted by hand, in their thousands, without even the benefits of a fan to cool the room. Fans would have blown the cards about!' (Page 46.)

Drs Daphne Christie and Tilli Tansey are to be congratulated for bringing together this remarkable group of experts who were involved in major developments in the treatment of tuberculosis over the second half of the twentieth century. The transcript will prove an invaluable document for future historians of tuberculosis and of medicine.

Linda Bryder

University of Auckland

SHORT-COURSE CHEMOTHERAPY FOR TUBERCULOSIS

The transcript of a Witness Seminar held by the Wellcome Trust Centre for the History of Medicine at UCL, London, on 3 February 2004

Edited by D A Christie and E M Tansey

SHORT-COURSE CHEMOTHERAPY FOR TUBERCULOSIS

Participants

Dr Joseph Angel
Sir Christopher Booth
Dr Ian Campbell
Sir Iain Chalmers
Dr Kenneth Citron
Sir John Crofton
Professor Janet Darbyshire
Dr Peter Davies
Dr Freda Festenstein
Mrs Gaye Fox*
Dr David Girling (Chair)
Professor Alan Glynn
Professor John Grange
Dr Elizabeth Hills
Dr Tony Jenkins
Dr Amina Jindani
Dr Adrian Martineau
Dr Jeanette Meadway
Professor Denis (Denny) Mitchison
Dr John Moore-Gillon
Professor Andrew Nunn
Professor Lawrence (Peter) Ormerod
Dr Knut Øvreberg
Dr Geoff Scott
Dr Bertie Squire

Among those attending the meeting: Dr Gerry Davies, Dr Duncan Hutchison, Ms Ann Goodburn, Professor David Greenwood, Ms Ruth Hutt, Dr Owen McCarthy

Apologies include: Sir John Batten, Dr Shiu Lun Chan, Dr Jean Dickinson, Dr Andrew Douglas, Professor Jacques Grosset, Dr Alan Somner, Dr David Tyrrell†

*On behalf of Professor Wallace Fox

†Died 2 May 2005

Dr David Girling: Perhaps I can express a warm welcome to everybody to this witness seminar on short-course chemotherapy. It's good to see the interest that this topic has attracted. It's always seemed to me that a uniquely important feature of the development of short-course treatment has been the enormously large, worldwide programmes of randomized controlled trials, running in parallel with essential laboratory research. I think it has been those two components, complementing each other, that have been particularly important. Now sadly, of course, a notable absentee is Professor Wallace Fox (Figure 1),[1] although we are delighted that Gaye, his wife, is able to be here with us . As Director of the [British] Medical Research Council's Tuberculosis and Chest Diseases Unit,[2] Wallace was responsible for directing the crucial series of MRC clinical trials[3] that led to the development of the now internationally accepted six-month antituberculosis regimens, and it is indeed sad that his health no longer allows him to participate in events such as this. Perhaps we can all convey our affection and our very best wishes to him through Gaye. Our aim is that the style of this meeting should be informal. We are certainly invited to discuss and debate, but we are also invited to reminisce, to say what it was like at the time, and why things happened the way they did, the constraints that there were on the planning and the conduct of trials, and the laboratory work. So please remember the historical nature of today's seminar. Now is our chance to establish our role in history.[4]

We come to the first main topic: laboratory research and the integration of laboratory and clinical research. Denny Mitchison is kindly going to introduce this topic for us.

Professor Denis Mitchison: Thank you. One can think in terms of how fundamental the work was in the laboratory, and what was the timescale involved. If we take the most fundamental point, which is how the antibacterial drugs that we are concerned with, actually work, one finds that

---

[1] See biographical note on page 101 and Appendix 1 (page 75).

[2] Formerly the Tuberculosis Research Unit, 1946–68, the Tuberculosis and Chest Diseases Unit (TCDU) continued until the retirement of its director Professor Wallace Fox in 1986. Members included Tony Miller, Joan Heffernan, Bill Stott, Janet Darbyshire (Africa), David Girling (Hong Kong and Singapore), Ruth Tall, Peter Fayers and Andrew Nunn (statisticians).

[3] See Fox *et al.* (1999).

[4] Dr David Girling wrote: 'For a history of pulmonary tuberculosis, see Keers (1978). For a comprehensive review of the [British] Medical Research Council studies, see Fox *et al.* (1999).' Letter to Dr Daphne Christie, 28 July 2004. See also D'Arcy Hart (1946); Tansey and Reynolds (2000); Mitchison (2005).

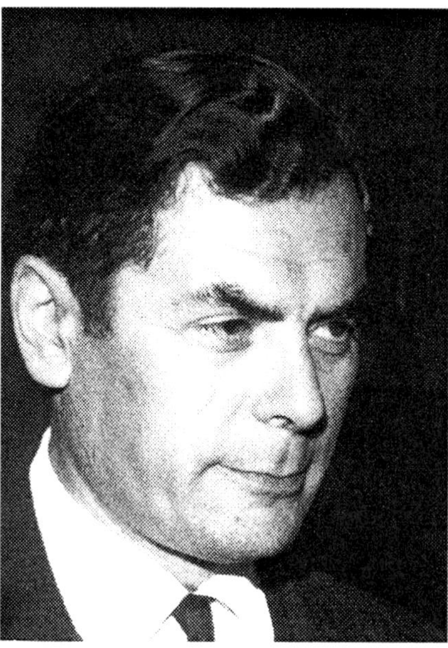

Figure 1: Professor Wallace Fox in 1959 at the time that he was working in India.

for rifampicin, its mode of action was known very early on in the 1960s.[5] This, with a little bit of addition, has not changed much since. But take the other almost as important drug, pyrazinamide. Pyrazinamide was introduced in 1952,[6] and it's only really in the last year or two that we have a clear idea of how it works. It is completely different from any other drug.[7] For that reason, one sometimes has to take a very long timescale. We used to look at pyrazinamide and say this is a drug that never behaves the same in two different experiments. Now the reasons for all that are much clearer.[8]

---

[5] Rifampicin facilitates treatment by means of its capacity to kill mycobacteria undergoing intermittent metabolism, the so-called 'sterilizing effect'. See note 34. For a reference to its biochemical mode of action, see Wehrli and Staehelin (1969).

[6] See Chorine (1945); McKenzie *et al.* (1948); See also Mitchison (1985); Fox *et al.* (1999); Zhang and Mitchison (2003).

[7] Zhang and Mitchison (2003). See also notes 19 and 22.

[8] Professor Denis Mitchison wrote: 'We did not understand that the degree of bacterial metabolism is as important as pyrazinamide concentration and pH in determining the bactericidal action of pyrazinamide.' Note on draft transcript, 22 March 2005.

The other aspect of fundamental research is to look at modelling in various ways. One can do it in terms of *in vitro* exposure of bacilli to drugs. For this, I would particularly think of Jean Dickinson's work on cultures and guinea-pigs, modelling intermittent administration of drugs, a very important component of modern treatment.[9] Also the immense importance of long-term mouse experiments, with the most recent ones done by Jacques Grosset in which the regimens model exactly those used in man.[10] Yet it has still to be proven that the results obtained would exactly simulate those in man. But there has been a huge change from very early crude tests in mouse experiments, to very exact simulation. So important is this that any change in regimens or drug treatment now has to be preceded by these long-term mouse experiments.

Girling: Denny, a thing I always found enormously helpful was your hypothesis on the different components of the bacterial population, because from the point of view of those of us who were actually running the trials, it has helped us to see how the various drugs of the regimen were active against, or sometimes had uniquely important actions against, certain components of the bacterial population.[11] Would you like to say a bit more about that?

Mitchison: This was a hypothesis put forward in about 1970. It started with the observation that if you look at what happens to the count of viable bacilli in sputum during treatment, you see an early abrupt fall and then it slows down.[12] This is quite different from the effects on a culture, where you get an exponential fall with a straight-line relationship between log count and time. This implies, I think, that there are at least two different bacterial populations. This idea led to the concept of a very early rapid killing of bacilli, mainly in the first two days of treatment, followed by a much slower killing of persisting organisms in what we call 'sterilizing' action. These two concepts are basic to an understanding of the action of drugs. If we could improve the speed of sterilizing by drugs, then we could shorten treatment. These ideas have been going on for the past 50 years.[13] The most recent paper on it, with Amina

---

[9] Intermittent treatment, that is treatment given twice or thrice weekly rather than daily. For a summary see Dickinson and Mitchison (1968, 1970); Mitchison and Dickinson (1971).

[10] Nuermberger *et al.* (2004a).

[11] Dr David Girling wrote: 'For an account of how laboratory and clinical research have complemented each other, see Girling (1989): 285–323.' Letter to Dr Daphne Christie, 28 July 2004.

[12] Mitchison (1979).

[13] Mitchison and Selkon (1956); Brindle *et al.* (2001).

Jindani and Caroline Doré, has looked in great detail at what happens during the first two days and then in the subsequent 12 days, and saw completely different drug actions during these two times.[14] But most important, it is in the search for new sterilizing drugs that one needs these particularly important ideas, because one needs methods for measuring sterilizing activity.[15] The bactericidal tests that you do on actively growing cultures are almost completely irrelevant. You need a completely different type of test to estimate how good at sterilizing are your drugs.

Sir John Crofton: You talked about new discoveries about just how pyrazinamide might work. Could you tell us what these are?

Mitchison: We go back to 1952 when pyrazinamide was first introduced, when you had this remarkable drug active in mice, not active at all in the test-tube, not active in guinea-pigs either. This drug was taken up rather fortuitously by Walsh McDermott at Cornell University, who started long-term animal experiments that showed that it went on killing bacteria when other drugs had stopped.[16] That was the essence of it. It was those experiments that actually led directly to the start of short-course regimens in man, as the initial clinical trial was started because of two series of mouse experiments: one at Cornell and the other at the Pasteur Institute.[17] For pyrazinamide the current idea is that it's a pro-drug: it gets converted to pyrazinoic acid, the active molecule. Pyrazinoic acid gets into the bacterial cell better in an acid environment, which is why pyrazinamide only acts in an acid environment. It then accumulates in the cell, because it's only excreted by an inefficient efflux pump and it's the accumulation of this acid that causes damage to cell membranes and eventually kills the cell. It doesn't have a site of action, as do other drugs, and the result is that the factors that influence its effect are completely different from other drugs. For instance, for all other drugs, as you slow down bacterial growth, the bactericidal effect gets less and less.[18] With pyrazinamide, it's exactly the opposite. As you slow down growth, so the efflux pump gets less efficient, the pyrazinoic acid accumulates and you get more bactericidal effect.[19]

---

[14] Jindani *et al.* (2003).

[15] Mitchison (2004).

[16] McCune *et al.* (1966).

[17] Grosset (1978).

[18] Dickinson and Mitchison (1981).

[19] For a review see Zhang and Mitchison (2003). See also notes 7 and 22.

Crofton: It seems you should not use it for the whole of the treatment, rather just at the beginning.[20]

Mitchison: Yes, the answer to that is that probably it has to have a slightly acid environment to work, and this is probably created by inflammation at the site of action. That dies down during treatment to leave a neutral environment in which the drug cannot act.[21] That's my hypothesis, but nobody else has got a better hypothesis.

Girling: In the clinical trials, we found that by giving pyrazinamide for the first two months that was enough, and you added nothing by giving it for longer, but that was just a pragmatic finding from the clinical side of the study.[22]

Crofton: Can I ask one other question? You mention about the mouse experiments for long term being so valuable. Isn't tuberculosis a bit different in the mouse – there are more intracellular organisms – and isn't it rather surprising that it parallels the human situation?

Mitchison: The most recent molecular studies suggest that both the nitric oxide expressed by immune cells, and low oxygen tension, which is the other controlling influence in preventing growth of tubercle bacilli, actually have similar controlling effects upon tubercle bacilli.[23] The changes in controlling gene expression patterns are closely similar, whether the bacilli are exposed to low oxygen tension or to nitric oxide. So, it may be that the immune process in the mouse cells, using nitric oxide, and low oxygen tension around extracellular bacilli in cavities, are having similar effects on the bacilli.

Girling: Amina, you were involved in part of the clinical side of this, this concept of looking at the bactericidal action of individual antituberculosis drugs. Would you like to tell us a bit about this? Was this in East Africa?

---

[20] Professor Denny Mitchison wrote: 'It is standard practice to prescribe pyrazinamide only in the initial two months of treatment. It is in the concluding phase of continuation treatment that pyrazinamide has been shown to be inactive in three different clinical trials.' Letter to Dr Daphne Christie, 9 May 2005. Sir John Crofton wrote: 'The laboratory experiments suggested that the drug would be effective for the whole of the treatment but the clinical research has shown that it was of little use over the first two months.' Letter to Dr Daphne Christie, 18 May 2005.

[21] See Mitchison (1985).

[22] Girling (1984).

[23] Voskuil *et al.* (2003).

Dr Amina Jindani: Yes, I was at that time coordinating the first short-course chemotherapy studies in East Africa, and this hypothesis of separate bacterial populations, and the drug having different effects on different bacterial populations, was very much around, and I had seen a publication saying that ethambutol in large doses, *in vitro*, increased the bacterial count.[24] Now this suggested to my simple mind that it caused the bacteria to divide and get them into an actively dividing state. So I had this wacky idea that if I could get the bacteria in my patients to divide in the lung, I could then zap them with rifampicin, cure their tuberculosis in two days, and win the Nobel Prize. Alas, we did a small study, using different doses of ethambutol and doing colony-forming counts, and that study showed no difference at all between the different doses of ethambutol. But we were visited at that time by two eminent gentlemen, Professor Wallace Fox and Professor Denny Mitchison, and because we were an MRC-collaborating unit they descended upon us from time to time.[25] I mentioned this small study to Denny and far from pouring scorn over it, he encouraged me to do the same counts on the rest of the drugs (these were in sputum, that is, counts of viable tubercle bacilli in the sputum). Yes, sputum of patients with active, newly diagnosed tuberculosis, and he helped me design the study, carry it through, and even wrote that famous paper that I think many of you know about.[26] But that's how the early bactericidal activity came into being.

Professor Alan Glynn: Denny, your results were in mice and in people, but of course mice vary enormously in their response to mycobacteria. Which strains were used mostly?[27]

Mitchison: The strain that is used is almost always the H37Rv strain. Historically that has been the strain most often studied. But there are studies done, particularly in the USA, with different strains, so it's not ideal. Now the point has been raised whether responses in mice are the same as those in man. In actual fact, most of the antituberculosis drugs penetrate into macrophages, into immune cells, fairly well. So you do in general tend to get much the same

---

[24] Dr Amina Jindani wrote: 'This was a conference abstract, which I cannot now trace.' Note on draft transcript, 23 March 2005.

[25] The East African Tuberculosis Investigation Centre, Nairobi, Kenya. The Director at the time was Dr Pierce Kent (see biographical note on page 103).

[26] Jindani *et al.* (1980). See also Donald *et al.* (2002).

[27] Professor Alan Glynn wrote: 'Strains of mice differ by two to three orders of magnitude in their innate resistance to mycobacteria. It would be surprising if this were not reflected in the results of chemotherapy.' Note on draft transcript, 10 June 2004. See Brown and Glynn (1987).

response. The only one which is a bit different is pyrazinamide, because pyrazinamide doesn't appear to be as bactericidal inside host, macrophage cells as it is outside, and so pyrazinamide in mouse tuberculosis, which is predominantly inside macrophages, is a much weaker drug than it seems to be in people.[28] But that doesn't usually make all that much difference to the experiment. I think it is quite remarkable how these long-term mouse experiments do correlate very closely with human disease, and there's been a very exciting recent study just published about moxifloxacin, which I think may disturb the whole future of chemotherapy, but that's again the present, not history.[29]

Girling: Anyone else like to say something on the laboratory side of the research, ask any further questions, or make comments?

Crofton: A minor one. When rifampicin was first found in Italy, a couple of people came over to me and said how should we try this out, because it's very difficult to feel that they could give it to patients who could have more well-established treatment, and it had to be given intravenously at that time.[30] I suggested that they gave the drug and did daily bacterial counts of sputum content for the first week or so, to make a preliminary test for bactericidal effect. The patients could then be switched to standard treatment. I am not quite sure whether they followed my advice. Someone else might know.

Dr John Moore-Gillon: Can I ask a very naive question and that is, what led you to look at these particular molecules? Things were clearly very different then from the way they are now, where pharmaceutical companies can screen literally thousands or tens of thousands of molecules to look at potential activity. What steered you in the direction of the drugs that we now have?

Mitchison: I seem to be asked to answer a lot of these questions. They occurred very largely by chance – apart from streptomycin, where there was good reason to look for a soil organism that produced an antibiotic like penicillin.[31] That was a very profitable way of looking for drugs. You had para-aminosalicylic acid (PAS) where the idea was that salicylic acid stimulated the metabolism of

---

[28] For mode of action of pyrazinamide see notes 7, 19 and 22.

[29] Professor Denis Mitchison wrote: 'Outbred "White Swiss" have been the strain of mice most often used, but balbc is also used.' Note on draft transcript, 22 March 2005. See Schurr *et al.* (1990); Nuermberger *et al.* (2004b).

[30] Sensi (1983). See page 10 and notes 34 and 72.

[31] See Waksman and Woodruff (1940); Schatz *et al.* (1944).

tubercle bacilli and hence an antagonist might be effective. But that turned out to be completely untrue, of course.[32] Then there was isoniazid,[33] which was a molecule similar to nicotinamide. Most of the other drugs started with nicotinamide. Again, nicotinamide acts much more like pyrazinamide, and completely unlike the action of isoniazid. So, you know, people followed clues, which were almost always wrong. The discovery of rifampicin, an antibiotic produced by soil *Streptomyces*, was a more logical process. You had pots of soil, hundreds of pots of soil from all over the world, and you looked at the soil *Streptomyces* to find your new drug. That worked like anything for a bit.[34]

Girling: Thank you very much. We can move to our next topic, which is the poor results of treatment achieved with standard long-term regimens in clinical practice. John Crofton has kindly agreed to introduce the topic.

Crofton: I am sorry this is going to be very anecdotal, but I think it's worth looking back to the beginning. Tuberculosis, before the drugs came in, was a notoriously relapsing disease. To begin with the aim of the new chemotherapies was only to try to arrest the disease, and the early MRC studies showed this very well. We had PAS/isoniazid and streptomycin at that time. Our group started work in 1952 in Edinburgh, just when isoniazid came in. We took part in the trials.[35] But to prevent relapse nobody knew how long to continue chemotherapy. We had found earlier on, when we had a couple of cases of primary PAS resistance who were initially given two drugs, including PAS, that by the time we had the lab results showing PAS resistance, the tuberculosis had become resistant to the second drug. We decided it was much safer to give all three available drugs initially and were surprised to find we were curing all new cases.[36]

---

[32] Erdei A (with comment by W E Snell) (1948). For a history of para-aminosalicylic acid, see Dubovsky (1988); see also Iseman (2002).

[33] Isoniazid (isonicotinic acid hydrazide – INAH) was first synthesized in 1912. In 1952 three isoniazid products were under trial in Britain: Rimifon, Roche; Nydrazid, Squibb; Pycazide, Herts Pharmaceuticals. See Anon (1952); McDermott (1952); Fox (1953).

[34] Rifampicin, one of 500 derivatives of rifamycin (introduced into therapy in 1968), was considered an improvement on the standard triple therapy of streptomycin, PAS and isoniazid, as it could be taken orally with improved antibacterial activity. See, for example, Saerens (1972); Garrod *et al.* (1973). For the nomenclature of the rifamycins, see Aronson (1999).

[35] Tuberculosis Chemotherapy Trials Committee (1952). See also Crofton (1954); Wallace *et al.* (1954).

[36] Crofton (1960); Ross *et al.* (1958).

But nobody knew how long to go on to prevent relapse. Naturally, some gave fairly short-term treatment to milder cases and long term to the really severe. J D (Ian) Ross looked at our relapse rate a year or two later. Paradoxically he found that it was the mild cases given short-term treatment who relapsed.[37] We had no relapses in those given 18 months or more.

At the same time we were doing a lot of surgery (lung resection), after preliminary chemotherapy, to prevent relapse, as was a widespread policy at that time.[38] Two of our research fellows, Derek Turnbull and Sheila Stewart, both I am afraid now dead, did multiple cultures of the resected specimens.[39] Their findings correlated very well with the relapse rates. For instance, in patients operated after 12–18 months' chemotherapy the relapse rate proved to be 1 per cent; cultures were positive in only 2 per cent. None of those who had had more than 18 months' treatment either relapsed or had positive cultures.[40] These relapse results were later confirmed by an MRC controlled trial of different lengths of chemotherapy in 'chronic' tuberculosis patients.[41] So 18 months became the standard duration.

How well this policy was adopted over the country in general, it's very difficult to know, because it really took about 20 years before everybody was given good treatment, so it was very difficult to judge the results. But the MRC did two studies, one in Scotland, and one in England and Wales, in which they looked at the total intake for a year and followed them up, but I cannot quite remember whether that was before or after triple therapy.[42] Perhaps somebody will be able to tell us that.

If we switch now to overseas, the early work by Denny [Mitchison] and Wallace Fox in Madras found that relapse rates, usually after a year of two-drug treatments, were relatively low, and that seemed a great financial advantage for Third World countries. As a result of this, they went on and did their

---

[37] Ross *et al.* (1958); See also Anon. (1977).

[38] See, for example, Pomerantz and Brown (1997).

[39] MacGregor *et al.* (1956).

[40] Crofton (1960). See also Ormerod and Prescott (2003).

[41] Medical Research Council/Tuberculosis Chemotherapy Trials Committee (1962).

[42] Spinaci (1990): 7–14.

wonderful work in East Africa, producing short-course chemotherapy. I hope they will be able to tell us what the routine results in those countries were in their previous studies, and in the general population, and perhaps they can do that more accurately for Singapore and Hong Kong, both of which had good services, but I cannot give those figures. My general impression, going round Third World countries was a 40 per cent cure rate, which most of them were getting. This seemed to improve dramatically with the short-course chemotherapy because there were fewer defaulters, but there were no accurate figures. As WHO showed, five to ten years ago the low cure rates in a number of countries resulted later in high rates of history of previous treatment in newly presenting patients, reflecting, of course, high rates of relapse and consequent drug resistance.[43] In contrast, well-supervised and completed therapy, short-course or long-term, both gave very low relapse rates.

Perhaps I could add one other thing? Short-course chemotherapy was initiated at a stage when the relevant drugs were very expensive. Accordingly, the Britain–Nepal Medical Trust,[44] with which I was involved, did a carefully controlled trial comparing results in two groups of remote hill districts that had previously had similar success rates using previously standard therapy.[45] If I remember correctly, it was 87 per cent success rate with short-course chemotherapy and 61 per cent with the other, so confirming the general impression that patients seemed to have much lower defaulter rate and thus did better with the short-course chemotherapy.

Professor Andrew Nunn: Just a couple of things. First, in relation to the poor results with standard chemotherapy. We did a number of surveys; Janet Darbyshire was more involved in these than I was. In the follow-up of the East African drug resistance surveys one of the striking things was the remarkable drop-off in the number of patients coming to collect their drugs. In the 1964 survey only 28 per cent of the patients were recorded as receiving drug supplies over the whole 12 months.[46]

---

[43] Spinaci (1990).

[44] The Britain–Nepal Medical Trust, a non-governmental organization, was set up in 1967 to help the people of Nepal and support the Tuberculosis Control Programmes. See Baker (1975). See also www.bnmt.org.np (visited 8 February 2005).

[45] Jochem *et al.* (1997).

[46] East African/[British] Medical Research Council Kenya Tuberculosis Follow-Up (1970).

The other thing I wanted to mention was a fascinating study we did in the Algerian Sahara where we were comparing two regimens: one a standard 12-month regimen, which was based on isoniazid/streptomycin/ethambutol; the other was a short-course, six-month rifampicin-based regimen.[47] The population included quite a lot of nomads who picked up their drugs at convenient places, or took sufficient supplies to get them from one place to another or to complete their treatment. The results in the short-course regimen were vastly better than in the standard treatment: 3 per cent compared with 17 per cent failures and relapses at two years. So it made an enormous difference that patients didn't actually have to go on taking their treatment for so long.

Professor Janet Darbyshire: Just after that, yes, we did surveys. The first one was before my time. I am not even sure if Amina [jindani] will remember it, but 1964, 1974 and 1984 in Kenya, and 1969, 1979, I think, in Tanzania.[48] And to me the striking find was the fact that you did quite well up to about six months, and I often wondered if that's why Wallace and Denny decided that the first big step into short-course chemotherapy was six months, because that's just about what you could get in people in East Africa.

Girling: Am I right in saying that these regimens included thiacetazone? Of course, in some communities, there was an enormous problem of thiacetazone toxicity wasn't there?

Darbyshire: Yes, thiacetazone is a fascinating drug. It's cheap, it's actually easier to combine with isoniazid and much easier to take than PAS–isoniazid which was probably the alternative at the time. But it seemed to be, again before my time, from all the wonderful studies that you did, it showed very interesting variations in its toxicity by population, which weren't really explained by ethnic group, or by anything in particular, but it was very well tolerated in East Africa. So that really formed the basis of the standard treatment of streptomycin plus thiacetazone and isoniazid (or thiazina as it was known), followed by thiacetazone and isoniazid alone.[49] But the fascinating thing is that I remember in the early 1980s, that all of a sudden we started to get quite

---

[47] Algerian Working Group/[British] Medical Research Council Cooperative Study (1984).

[48] See note 46. East African/[British] Medical Research Council (1977, 1979); Kenyan/[British] Medical Research Council (1989); Tanzanian/[British] Medical Research Council (1985).

[49] Thiazina – a combination of isoniazid and thiacetazone. See East African/[British] Medical Research Council (1970); Ipuge *et al.* (1995). See also Briggs *et al.* (1968).

severe Stevens–Johnson reactions to the thiacetazone, which was the serious skin side-effect.[50] We thought that maybe it was the wrong concentration, maybe there was something wrong with it, but in retrospect it was probably the very early cases of HIV infection. In people with HIV infection the incidence of adverse reactions is much higher, and the more severe reactions are common, hence most countries now are not using thiacetazone if they have a high incidence of HIV infection. So that's interesting. These probably were some of the early HIV infections in Africa.

Mitchison: Could I add a bit of evidence to this? The study reported by Pierce Kent, Wallace Fox and myself compared the thiacetazone regimens given in clinical trials with the results obtained in the survey.[51] Because what this showed was that although you could get excellent results with regimens in clinical trials, unfortunately when you looked at them in use in populations, the results were very much worse, and this was attributed to failure to take drugs in the latter months of treatment.

Dr Peter Davies: I'm really a newcomer to this. It's really what Sir John was glossing over, and it's something that I have had in the back of my mind for 20 years and I have been meaning to ask. There is very good literature on streptomycin alone and also on streptomycin against streptomycin and PAS, but I am at a loss to find anything very good on streptomycin and PAS, against streptomycin and PAS and isoniazid. Were there any randomized controlled trials done on those two comparisons?

Mitchison: The first trials were with streptomycin and PAS and streptomycin and isoniazid, weren't they?

Davies: No, they did streptomycin/isoniazid versus PAS/isoniazid, but not streptomycin/PAS, you see that was never included.

Mitchison: That was a matter of great interest because streptomycin is not a very good drug, it's only moderately good, whereas on the whole isoniazid is an excellent drug, and you see this on the very rare occasions when a comparison of that sort is made. It was actually made in some of the US studies, but the method of analysis doesn't help you very much because it was never really very clear how well those regimens did. Then there was a very

---

[50] For a review see Ferguson *et al.* (1971). See also Harland (1962); Hussain *et al.* (1973).

[51] Kent *et al.* (1970).

small study done in Bulawayo comparing streptomycin/thiacetazone with thiacetazone/isoniazid, in which the streptomycin/thiacetazone did extremely badly.[52] So I think there is no doubt that streptomycin is not actually the world's best drug; nor is PAS, everybody agrees on that.

Davies: I would like to be absolutely clear about this. So there has been no study done, as you might have expected, of streptomycin plus PAS, which are the oldest two, against this newcomer isoniazid, and you might have given streptomycin and PAS and isoniazid, the old against the new, it's never been done.

Mitchison: It has in the USA, but the methods of assessment are very different from those we would use now and so it is actually very difficult to assess the relative merits of those two. If you like I could try to give you a reference to it.[53]

Davies: But this seemed to be a big slip up on the part of the MRC who started well but didn't continue logically.

Professor John Grange: Peter has just asked a question that has been bothering him for 20 years. May I do likewise and ask our experts when, how and why did isoniazid monotherapy get introduced for treating latent tuberculosis? The reason I ask is that I have always been puzzled by a paradox, which nobody has explained: isoniazid, as we know from the work of Mitchison and others, hits the actively replicating mycobacteria, and yet we assume that in latent tuberculosis these organisms are dormant. So it seems illogical. How does it work and why?

Dr Joseph Angel: A brief historical memory. Isoniazid exploded on to the tuberculosis scene and seeing the excellent results that were produced by using it alone, there was no question of leaving it out of any clinical trial.

Grange: I suspect that helps to answer Peter Davies's question. This was before there were any ideas of different bacterial populations, and so presumably drugs, including isoniazid, were classified as either effective or not effective. Am I right in thinking that isoniazid appeared on the scene fairly soon after PAS?

---

[52] Briggs *et al.* (1968).

[53] Medical Research Council (1955); Tucker (1955); International Union Against Tuberculosis (1964). See also Donald *et al.* (2002).

Crofton: In point of fact, PAS was developed before.[54] It wasn't published before. It was being used in Sweden before. Can I just tell a story about the early isoniazid? You remember Walsh McDermott was one of the people who did the first testing of isoniazid and he thought that isoniazid-resistant organisms didn't matter.[55] When patients produced resistant organisms and these were injected into guinea-pigs they proved less pathogenic. He sold this to WHO. Monotherapy with isoniazid was the cheap answer to Third World tuberculosis. Everybody tries to forget it nowadays. Walsh and I had tremendous, if good-tempered battles, but for a number of years monotherapy was used in many countries and caused a great deal of isoniazid resistance, both primary and secondary.[56] Of course monotherapy with isoniazid, as a preventive for tuberculin-positive individuals without disease, proved very effective in North America and resulted in little resistance.

Dr Ian Campbell: I came into respiratory medicine in 1970, so I am a relatively new boy in this audience. But I came in when 18 months' PAS and isoniazid with three months' streptomycin was standard treatment, and used until 1975 when the British Thoracic Association's (BTA) trials were published.[57] I have been in respiratory medicine since, and everyone has been talking about high relapse rates with 18 months' PAS/isoniazid, three months' streptomycin, especially overseas. I don't know about my other colleagues of similar vintage, of whom there are some about still. Had there been a high relapse rate in Britain in standard practice? Has Janet [Darbyshire] any data on this from the survey she did before? Because it seemed to me that it worked in Britain quite well. Now that's anecdotal and I didn't conduct any surveys.

Dr Kenneth Citron: If you cast your mind back to the 1960s and 1970s, we had many tuberculosis nurses, we had well-staffed clinics, and therefore we could monitor self-administered drugs extremely efficiently. I ran a large chest clinic in Wandsworth, south London, in the 1960s and early 1970s. At that time we were giving isoniazid/PAS for at least 18 months and often for two years, with streptomycin added in the initial three months. In 1971 we

---

[54] Lehmann (1946); Dubovsky (1988).

[55] McDermott (1969).

[56] Drug-resistant tuberculosis can be transmitted (primary) or develop during the course of treatment (secondary). Mitchison *et al.* (1957); McDermott (1970).

[57] British Thoracic and Tuberculosis Association (1975).

published our results.[58] In routine treatment, we found that 90 per cent of our patients had completed the prescribed treatment. Of the 10 per cent that didn't, most of them had died, mostly from nontuberculous causes, mostly elderly men. Among the 90 per cent who completed treatment, all but 2 per cent became culture negative. We had a post-treatment follow-up for between three and seven years, and found that none had relapsed. I can tell you that we were delighted with the results of long-course therapy at that time. But adequate staffing and meticulous attention to detail were needed to attain good results.

Moore-Gillon: To put myself in a historical context, I am even younger than Ian Campbell. I qualified in 1976, so was training as a clinical student in the mid-1970s, and then in respiratory medicine from 1980 onwards. I want to come back to the question of isoniazid monotherapy for latent tuberculosis. For those who were there at the time, how much of it was a pragmatic decision, in that you had a patient who was clinically well but you were telling them that they had a potential problem, and when they asked you, 'What can you do about it?', you had to reply, 'Well, you can have two or three months of injections, that will make you very dizzy, and some disgusting tasting granules, or you can take this fairly simple and benign medication.' In practical terms, you could persuade people to take isoniazid, whereas you couldn't persuade them to take combination therapy for latent tuberculosis. Was that a factor?

Crofton: In the early stages people with minor lesions were usually very carefully watched until they broke down. We persuaded our colleagues in Scotland, with some hesitation I think, to randomize these patients into doing the normal follow-up or having PAS and isoniazid, and we showed a very significant difference.[59] This was an all-Scottish study. However, that was using the two drugs. I was always worried about resistance, with the single drug, and when they did this North American study, they did get a few, but it was only one or two. It was quite a small resistance risk.

Mitchison: The study of isoniazid in chemoprophylaxis was done on a massive scale by the US Public Health Service.[60] They went into the question of whether it caused isoniazid resistance and concluded it did not. You got a little

---

[58] Citron and de Silva (1971); See also Citron (1972, 1988).

[59] Scottish Thoracic Society (1963).

[60] Ferebee (1970).

selection of those people who started off with isoniazid-resistant strains, because the chemoprophylaxis wouldn't work in them, but I think they felt that, as you needed about 10^5 sensitive organisms to have one mutant bacillus resistant to isoniazid, you simply don't get that number of organisms or anything like it in dormant disease. Of course it is quite a different matter in treating people with active disease and you have to screen them very carefully.

Girling: It seems to me that the message that comes across from this section of the meeting is that those old long-term regimens were actually quite effective regimens, and that the main problem in their use in routine clinical conditions was patient compliance, their actual compliance in treatment. And so there was great pressure to look for regimens that could be given under full supervision for a much shorter period of time, maybe with some intermittency, and not just daily administration. We turn now to the importance of the combination of isoniazid/rifampicin/pyrazinamide.

Darbyshire: I will kick off, although I am introducing something that again started before I joined the MRC Tuberculosis and Chest Diseases Unit in 1974. I think the first step in establishing the importance of rifampicin and pyrazinamide was 'Study R', which was the really quite radical study, that looked at three drug combination (triple combination therapy) of streptomycin and isoniazid with rifampicin, with pyrazinamide, and with thiacetazone, as well as streptomycin and isoniazid alone, all given for six months, and compared with the standard East African regimen.[61] That very clearly showed that the two drugs that were really potent were rifampicin and pyrazinamide, in addition to the streptomycin and isoniazid. So that, I think, was the foundation and I believe it was really Amina Jindani, Pierce Kent and Joan Heffernan, who were responsible for overseeing that trial. That was really the beginning. After that, what followed was an unbelievably elegant series of studies, crossing continents and crossing countries, which showed the important role of these drugs, both in the initial phase, and all the way through, and I can never decide whether I drew the short straw or the long straw, because I inherited East Africa from Joan, which meant I had fantastic elephants and lions, and spent hours and hours in Land Rovers. David [Girling] actually was very lucky – he got to go to Hong Kong and Singapore.

It seems to me that in East Africa we had the studies where it was very clear at that stage, that we couldn't give rifampicin and pyrazinamide for six months;

---

[61] Jindani (1976).

they were just too expensive, and actually you couldn't give streptomycin for six months, it was too painful. At that time we were keeping the patients in hospital too, which again is not really feasible. So that's really how we moved into the initial intensive phase of four-drug treatment – streptomycin/isoniazid/pyrazinamide/rifampicin – followed by a cheap combination phase. All the studies in East Africa were focusing around: firstly establishing whether pyrazinamide was important in that first two-month phase – which it clearly was – if we took it away, if we could drop to one month, which would have been even better, but it wasn't as good; and secondly, looking at the combination phase afterwards. But that was paralleled by studies which, as I say, you, David, were 'minding', and Andrew probably knows more about, so that's perhaps the next step.

Nunn: I would like to say a little bit more about East Africa before we go on to Hong Kong. The study, which was affectionately known as Study R, had a fascinating design, because it answered so many questions and provoked so many hypotheses. Janet [Darbyshire] mentioned the fact that patients were in hospital for the full six months, and that was intentional, in order to give the maximum opportunity to see if these drugs worked and how well they worked. One thing that should also be said, of course, was the cost of rifampicin in those days. It was between £100 and £200 for six months, a very expensive drug at that time. Ethically it would have been very difficult to do a trial like that today. We are seeing antiretrovirals coming into Africa now for HIV/AIDS, but that's only because the drugs have been considerably reduced in cost. Prior to that reduction, many ethicists would have considered trials of HIV drugs quite inappropriate in such a setting.

I mentioned the cost of rifampicin, which was between four and ten times as expensive as pyrazinamide, so when the first study was planned in Hong Kong it was decided not to study rifampicin, but to base the study on pyrazinamide. Because the results of pyrazinamide were not as good as those of rifampicin, two durations were compared: six months and nine months. The six-month results were considerably inferior to results in East Africa. This is something that we have seen over the years too: the results in East Africa differ from results in Hong Kong. Certainly you cannot give the same drugs and get the same results necessarily, unless the regimens are highly effective. So the first study in Hong Kong investigated only streptomycin, isoniazid and pyrazinamide, looking at intermittent as well as daily regimens.[62]

---

[62] Hong Kong Chest Service/[British] Medical Research Council (1977, 1979). See also Horsfall (1973).

The second study in Hong Kong actually did include rifampicin and, in fact, both the second study in East Africa, along with the second study in Hong Kong, brought together the three drugs, isoniazid, rifampicin and pyrazinamide for the first time. The striking finding was a dramatic increase in the culture conversion rates by two months, compared with any other regimens. From that point onwards those three drugs pretty well stayed together, although both the second and the third short-course studies in Hong Kong included a comparison of ethambutol substituted for pyrazinamide; ethambutol was clearly inferior.[63]

Darbyshire: Study X (the fourth short-course study in East Africa) was actually great.[64] We wouldn't be allowed to do it today, but Andrew and I used to analyse it about once a week, to see how many relapses there were, because this was the study that actually showed that you don't need to carry pyrazinamide all the way through. I think it was this study (Study X in Africa) and a corresponding study in Singapore that really showed that what is now virtually a standard regimen – of streptomycin/isoniazid/rifampicin/pyrazinamide, followed by isoniazid and rifampicin – was just as good as carrying on with the pyrazinamide all the way through. So I think that was an important study. The reason we watched it very carefully was that we found out if you dropped to four months, which is what we hoped we could, you actually have very high relapse rates. So we learnt a lot about the minimum duration of chemotherapy, with probably the most potent combination we had at that time, and probably still have today.

Jindani: I want to tell you about two completely different aspects of study R, which was the first short-course chemotherapy study that I had the privilege of coordinating in 42 centres in East Africa and Zambia. The first is this business about informed consent.[65] Of course there were no 20-page consent forms to be signed, and it would have been difficult to get African patients with tuberculosis to sign a 20-page form; they might have signed it, but they might not have understood it. I did it this way: when they came to the hospital, I would say, 'Look you have tuberculosis, if I give you treatment for 18 months, and you take it, you will be cured. But we have drugs that we want

---

[63] Hong Kong Chest Service/[British] Medical Research Council (1979, 1987).

[64] East African/[British] Medical Research Council (1978).

[65] The process by which a patient can make an informed decision about his/her wish to participate in a trial.

to test on you, and we think six months of treatment will be enough if we give you those drugs. But for that you will have to come into hospital and remain in hospital for six months. Can you do it? Or can't you do it'? I think that was a pretty good way of getting informed consent from them, because those who couldn't stay, didn't stay. Now the second point is about the giraffes and the elephants. No! Tigers. All I remember after a site visit, was the car going off the road and myself going through the windscreen and ending up at the bottom of the Rift Valley and having to have my face reconstructed after that, so I think, Janet [Darbyshire], you were pretty lucky.

Girling: It seems to me that you have brought up an enormously important issue about informed consent, because it sometimes bothered me whether these trials could even be conducted today just on that basis. In Hong Kong and Singapore, Wallace, or Wallace and I, would go over and discuss the plans for a trial with the Minister of Health, and with the Director of the National Tuberculosis Service. If they were happy with the trial, and you had to persuade them, they had to be convinced that this was a trial that was relevant to their country, and sometimes plans of trials had to be changed on the basis of what they said. But in a sense that was where the major step of informed consent occurred. Patients certainly were told that they were in a trial, because in Hong Kong and Singapore we did occasionally get a patient who decided not to take part, but they were very few and far between. This does actually raise quite an important issue: the whole aspect of informed consent, and if anyone would like to contribute on that, we would be very interested to know.

Mitchison: Before we get on to that, which I think is a side issue for the moment, let us go back to Study R, because I think it's important to realize why Study R was done. I was at the first meeting where the planning of this study was made, with Andrew, but David, I can't remember were you there? [No, I don't think so.] And Janet certainly was not. We were going there to plan a new study in East Africa, and they came quite often. Wallace turned up and he really sprang a bombshell on us, because he said he had been talking to Georges Canetti,[66] who was firmly convinced from the mouse experiments that he had done that rifampicin was a wonder drug that could be used to shorten treatment.[67] That really was the reason why Study R got started. I added in the

[66] Grumbach *et al.* (1969); Professor Georges Canetti (1911–71) was at the IUAT and Institut Pasteur in Paris [see Grosset (1971)].

[67] See, for example, McDermott *et al.* (1954).

fact that I had been in contact with Walsh McDermott and his mouse experiments on pyrazinamide for many years.[68] As a result, we also included pyrazinamide, which nobody else had thought of at all at the time. It was the mouse work, at Cornell and the Pasteur Institute in Paris, that led to short-course chemotherapy.

Having said that, I perhaps should also say that, as I understood it, the physicians in Hong Kong were at first dead against this dangerous drug, pyrazinamide, which they associated with liver damage.[69] It was only with some difficulty that the plans for the first study with pyrazinamide and no rifampicin were put in place, but as soon as the results came through, no study was complete without pyrazinamide. So I think there was a radical change of opinion.

Crofton: The reason was that when pyrazinamide was used early on, it was given in much bigger doses, and that's when they got this disastrous liver damage.

Campbell: When we were running the second BTA [British Thoracic Association] trial in the UK, which included pyrazinamide, the fear of the organizing committee, which included Ken Citron, Joe Angel and Joe Selkon, was that physicians would not want to put patients in, because physicians in Britain in the middle 1970s were still scared of pyrazinamide. I think it was to the credit of the BTA members that they grasped the nettle. Consent by patients was not as informed as it would be today, because all we did for those trials was to say to the patients, 'Look, we are running a study of four different durations of tuberculosis treatment that you used to have to take for such a long time, and we are going to try to see if we can shorten it, would you take part?' And the patients uniformly said, 'Yes'.

Angel: I would like to go back a little while, just to talk about the genesis of the BTA trials. My interest was first aroused by going to a BTA meeting in Cambridge in 1969, when a Belgian physician, Dr Gyselen [André Gyselen], described the results of a three-month treatment with the three regimens, which I have given the details of in the sheet you have in front of you (Figure 2).[70] Ethambutol plus isoniazid, ethambutol plus rifampicin, and rifampicin plus isoniazid, and you will see that at the end of the three months of

---

[68] See, for example, McCune *et al.* (1966).

[69] See Hong Kong Tuberculosis Treatment Services/[British] Medical Research Council (1976).

[70] See Gyselen and Simon-Porthier (1969): 328; Gyselen (1994).

Regimen	Number of patients	Culture-negative at three months
Rifampicin/Isoniazid	29	28
Rifampicin/Ethambutol	30	29
Ethambutol/Isoniazid	27	22

Figure 2: Sputum conversion in advanced pulmonary tuberculosis on treatment with three regimens of chemotherapy.

Dr Joseph Angel wrote: 'In the long-term chemotherapy study conducted by the MRC with streptomycin for six weeks/PAS/isoniazid or PAS/isoniazid, culture negativity rates at three months were 55 and 44 per cent respectively.' Note on Figure 2, 3 February 2004. Adapted from Gyselen and Simon-Porthier (1969): 328.

Regimen	Number of patients	Months					
		1	2	3	4	5	6
SHRZ (six months)	146	38	77	97	99	100	100
EHRZ (six months)	141	33	77	99	99	100	100
EHR (nine months)	157	29	64*	88*	98	100	100

S=Streptomycin; H=Isoniazid; R=Rifampicin; Z=Pyrazinamide; E=Ethambutol

Figure 3: Cumulative percentage of patients culture-negative at each month during the course of drug treatment.

* Significant reduction in sputum conversion in non-pyrazinamide containing-regimen. Adapted from British Thoracic Association. (1981) A controlled trial of six months chemotherapy in pulmonary tuberculosis. First Report: Results during chemotherapy. *British Journal of Diseases of the Chest* **75**:141–53.

chemotherapy, the sputum conversion rates were significantly higher with the two rifampicin-containing regimens, and much higher than with the PAS–isoniazid regimen, which was standard at that time.

So I thought about this for a year or two, and by this time I was on the Research Committee of the BTA, so I put it to the Research Committee that we might consider doing a trial of reduced durations. Initially, it provoked a little hesitation, not surprisingly because most of the members of the committee had spent their professional lives encouraging people to take drugs for longer and longer periods. It had gone up from six weeks to three months, to six months, to 18 months, to two years. So there was quite a lively discussion as to the ethics of this trial, but some of us stood out, in particular Alan Somner,[71] who, I am sorry to see, wasn't able to come to this meeting. As a result of his intervention the committee said, 'OK, those who are enthusiastic about it, should go away, form a subcommittee and plan the trial.' And so we did. We arranged that we were going to put it to the summer meeting of the BTA in June 1972. It was interesting that at the second meeting of the Research Committee, when we put forward our protocols, the mood had changed completely. People who were originally rather sceptical were all for it and made very positive suggestions. We didn't know anything about the East African studies, and we only learnt about them I think, about three weeks before this June meeting, and you have just heard the results of the East African study, so that encouraged us enormously. So we set out the protocol at a special meeting of the clinicians who might be involved where they turned up in droves and were extremely enthusiastic. They clearly didn't like the standard 18-month or two-year regimens, and were only too delighted to participate in a trial of shorter durations, and in fact this was reflected in the large number of patients submitted for the study, which was 911 in seven months and, as Ian Campbell probably remembers, taxed us to the utmost.

This study was funded by two pharmaceutical companies, Ciba-Geigy (Basel) and Lepetit (Milan), and was launched in October 1972.[72] We compared four durations, six, nine, 12 and 18 months of rifampicin plus isoniazid with the first two months being allocated at random to either streptomycin or ethambutol, with follow-up for five years. The results were quite striking. Only one patient still had positive sputum cultures at the end of chemotherapy. The relapse rates were 7 per cent for the six-month group, and 1.7 per cent for the nine-month group, which occurred very late in the follow-up, 1 per cent in the 12-month group and none in the 18-month group. On the strength of these

---

[71] Alan Somner collaborated with Joe Angel in running the BTA/BTS studies. See, for example, Somner (1975); Angel *et al.* (1976).

[72] Dr Joseph Angel wrote: 'Lepetit Research Laboratories in Milan developed rifampicin and were extremely helpful in the planning of the first BTA study. They were later absorbed into Dow Chemicals, which is now, I think, Merrill-Dow. The details of the study are given above.' Letter to Dr Daphne Christie, 7 April 2005. See Kradolfer (1968a, 1968b); Sensi (1983).

results, the BTA recommended a regimen of rifampicin plus isoniazid for nine months, supplemented by ethambutol, because we had more trouble with streptomycin toxicity than ethambutol toxicity, in a dose of 25 mg per kg for the first two months.[73]

Girling: Thank you very much. There are two points that occurred to me that come out of this. I think it is important to emphasize the extraordinarily important international scope of these trials. There were MRC trials, but other groups were conducting trials as well. I have listed the countries that I thought were involved, and you can probably think of others. There were those in East and Central Africa, Hong Kong, Singapore, Transkei, Poland, what was then East Germany, Czechoslovakia, Algeria, Finland, Argentina, as well as, of course, the UK and France; and, yes the Korea spinal tuberculosis studies, that's right. Also the collaboration of the pharmaceutical industry was essential. We were hoping to get somebody from the pharmaceutical industry here, but unfortunately have not been successful.[74] It really does emphasize how important the collaboration of the pharmaceutical industry was in conducting certainly the MRC programme and evidently other programmes as well.

Sir Iain Chalmers: I have a question about funding of this very impressive series of controlled trials. It arises from something that I think I understood Wallace Fox[75] to say at a meeting in 1986 at the London Hospital, which was convened by the Consumers' Association to discuss clinical trials in society. My understanding is that the manufacturers of antituberculosis drugs contributed to a research fund, which was then administered by the MRC to do whichever studies seemed to be most important. Have I mis-remembered something that Wallace said?

Mitchison: The point was that in the early days the drugs were provided free from the manufacturers and at the time this was the only contribution that they made. The actual running of the studies and of the units concerned was

---

[73] For a description of streptomycin's toxicity and side-effects, see, for example, Barber and Garrod (1963): 98–101.

[74] Dr David Girling wrote: 'Pharmaceutical companies provided free drugs for numerous randomized trials. They also contributed to *per diem* payments enabling collaborators from developing countries to attend meetings and conferences, and sponsored some useful research meetings.' Letter to Dr Daphne Christie, 8 April 2005. See Herxheimer *et al.* (1986).

[75] See biographical note on page 101 and Appendix 1.

entirely MRC-funded. At a much later stage, there began to be this ancillary fund which was actually only a quite minor contribution made by drug companies, and particularly by the manufacturers of rifampicin who provided a great deal of support.[76] This was used for various ancillary purposes, including often some support of the local tuberculosis programmes in the countries concerned.

Girling: Perhaps I can finish this discussion by emphasizing again what a huge achievement was made by this large programme of randomized clinical trials in the various countries. This programme determined clinically the best drug combinations to use, the appropriate duration for treatment, both in the daily initial phase and in the continuation phase. It determined that pyrazinamide need be given for no more than two months. It determined appropriate drug dosages in both phases of treatment. It identified regimens that were both highly active and yet relatively free of adverse effects. It produced regimens that could be given under full supervision, or with very high levels of supervision, and that were robust in the face of some lack of compliance. It produced regimens for which there was minimal risk of the development of acquired resistance during chemotherapy and failure, and with very low relapse rates after treatment. I think this is probably one of the largest international combined research enterprises that have been conducted in the history of medicine.

Campbell: I would like to say that it wasn't driven by pharmaceutical companies, which have driven the beta-blockade research, the H_2 antagonist research, the inhaled steroid research and other fields, ever since.[77] It came from within the profession and the research organizations.

Girling: Thank you very much. Shall we now move on to consider the recommended short-course regimens?[78]

Darbyshire: A lot of the importance of the programme of research, which was involving collaborators in so many countries and so many different conditions, was actually to produce not just one recommended regimen, but regimens that were widely applicable in many different circumstances. With my East African hat on, what we wanted was something that was cheap, that didn't actually

---

[76] Professor Denis Mitchison wrote: 'Wallace Fox administered the product. The main support for all of the work came from the Medical Research Council and the Overseas Development Agency (the Department for International Development since 1997).' Note on draft transcript, 22 March 2005.

[77] See, for example, Reynolds and Tansey (2001); Christie and Tansey (2002).

[78] International Union Against Tuberculosis and Lung Disease (1988).

require patients to be in hospital all the time, and that was relatively nontoxic. So the regimen that came out of this programme as the recommended regimen that was widely adopted by the IUATLD (International Union Against Tuberculosis and Lung Disease)[79] and the WHO was an eight-month regimen, of two months of streptomycin/isoniazid/rifampicin/pyrazinamide, followed by six months' thiacetazone and isoniazid. That extra two months was shown in a study whose name I cannot remember, but I think it was Study U, to really make a difference compared with just stopping at six months. So that was very widely introduced. There were quite a lot of debates as to whether the first two months should be fully supervised and therefore required hospital admission, and some quite, I won't say angry debates, but noisy debates, particularly between Karel Styblo and Wallace occurred. But I think that was the big contribution that the African studies made, a widely used regimen. The impact of HIV has meant that a lot of people have switched over from thiacetazone to ethambutol, although until very recently we never tested that regimen and Amina might like to say something about that.

Jindani: As Janet said, the recommended regimen then became isoniazid/rifampicin/pyrazinamide supplemented by streptomycin in the initial intensive phase, followed by thiacetazone/isoniazid in the continuation phase for six months. Now, with the arrival of the HIV pandemic, people did not want to give streptomycin, so they have replaced streptomycin with ethambutol.[80] The basis of this was the second BTA study, which showed that when you gave streptomycin and the other three drugs, followed by isoniazid/rifampicin, the relapse rates were 0.8 per cent. But when you replaced the streptomycin with ethambutol, the relapse rate was 2.4 per cent, and that was, I think, accepted as equivalent, although it is three times higher than when giving streptomycin.

The other assumption that is made by the tuberculosis world, especially by WHO and the IUATLD, is that thiacetazone could equally be replaced by

---

[79] The International Union Against Tuberculosis (IUAT) began as the International Conference for Tuberculosis Doctors in 1867. In 1902 the Central Bureau for the Prevention of Tuberculosis was housed in Berlin and became Paris based in 1920, as the International Union Against Tuberculosis. In 1986, a mandate extended its function to include other lung diseases such as asthma and tobacco complaints. For further details see www.tbrieder.org/ (site visited 19 April 2005). See also Enarson (1995).

[80] Dr Amina Jindani wrote: 'Streptomycin is given by injection and there is a risk of transmission of HIV if the same needle is used in more than one patient.' Note on draft transcript, 23 March 2005.

ethambutol in the continuation phase, but this combination, although recommended, was never tried in a clinical trial. We have recently just completed such a clinical trial, and the results when compared with the six-month regimen, rifampicin, in the continuation phase, showed that ethambutol/isoniazid for eight months was not as good as the rifampicin and isoniazid.[81] So now we are back to another, or several, probably noisy debates, because the big question now is with the arrival of antiretrovirals in Africa, should we give rifampicin in the continuation phase, or should we not give rifampicin in the continuation phase. It will be interesting to hear what anybody else might have to say on that.

Darbyshire: Just to pick up on that. One of the problems is the interaction between rifampicin and many of the anti-HIV drugs, which I think has led to quite a lot of debate as to whether you start the tuberculosis treatment first, or start the antiretroviral treatment, so I think there are huge numbers of issues now around the management of what is a major problem, namely coinfection with HIV and tuberculosis worldwide, but particularly in sub-Saharan Africa.

Crofton: Can I ask a question? I know the IUATLD was very worried about using ethambutol or rifampicin in the follow-up phase in developing countries, because they thought it wouldn't be taken properly and there would be much more resistance. Have you any evidence of increased resistance as a result of either of these two uses, compared with before when they weren't being used in the follow-up phase?

Jindani: There is one report from Tanzania about increased resistance to rifampicin, but really it has never been confirmed.[82] The IUATLD is still very much wedded to thiacetazone, but in sub-Saharan Africa I think that they will have to change. The latest recommendations still say thiacetazone/isoniazid, but as I have said the great debate now is whether we should give rifampicin/isoniazid, because you have a shorter duration of treatment, and you have a higher cure rate. That debate has only just started. And Andrew reminds us there is no cost problem.

Moore-Gillon: One of the things a political historian, if not the medical historian, might like to pick up on, is the mention of the involvement of East Germany, Czechoslovakia and Poland. That's a quite extraordinary thing, it

---

[81] Jindani *et al.* (2004).

[82] Chonde (1980).

seems to me. One can understand how many other parts of the world were involved. But you are dealing with countries behind the Iron Curtain at that time. Maybe it was heading up for the Prague spring in Czechoslovakia. How on earth did you manage it?

Crofton: I went to Poland in about 1956, but their system there was that they had one major postgraduate training centre for tuberculosis. The head of that unit, Professor Marion Zierski of Lodz, spent quite a long time with us in Edinburgh and went back convinced about the ordinary good chemotherapy. Under the communist regime, all chest physicians had to attend a revision course in Zierski's unit every five years. So it was very easy to spread a good chemotherapy regimen quite quickly. Then they went on to do their own trials.[83]

Mitchison: Can I make one further comment about this problem of resistance? What happened in Amina's study is what you expect. You start with initial isoniazid resistance and that's roughly between 8 and 9 per cent or so of many populations, as in much of East Africa. If you continue such patients with an ethambutol/isoniazid regimen in the continuation phase, then you get quite a high percentage of failures occurring. I cannot remember what the figures are, but I would give it at about 17 per cent or something like that. If you have a six-month rifampicin/isoniazid continuation, it makes no difference whatsoever, because isoniazid is not doing anything in the six-month regimen; we could leave it out perfectly well.

Campbell: I want to pop back to streptomycin versus ethambutol, which was I think quite a critical comparison. Amina [Jindani] says that ethambutol was inferior to streptomycin, but in fact, and I will seek Joe's and Tony's memories on this, and Ken's, in the two BTA trials we showed no difference between the ethambutol- and the streptomycin-containing initial regimens.[84] So in the British population anyway, there was no difference. But turn it round. We are all doctors and medically orientated scientists in here. The patients were delighted to hear and to consider that they didn't have to have two or three months of injections, but they could possibly take two or three months of tablets, and I suspect that if there was any difference in the relapse rate, the patients would have said, 'I still want the tablets, I will take my chance'.

---

[83] Sir John Crofton wrote: 'The same year Noel Rist and I were invited to the Central Research Institute in Prague (Professor Jancik) where we had a similar effect.' Letter to Dr Daphne Christie, 28 June 2004. See Snider *et al.* (1986).

[84] British Thoracic and Tuberculosis Association. (1975); see also Somner (1975); Angel *et al.* (1976).

Angel: I have got the paper here [British Thoracic Association (1982)], the relapses were, two out of 119 (1.7 per cent) with the initial streptomycin, four out of 127 (3.2 per cent) in the initial ethambutol and there were two out of 127 (1.6 per cent) with the new standard regimen without pyrazinamide in the second BTA trial (the nine-month regimen).[84a]

The other point I would like to make about the second BTA trial, is that although there was, as Ian [Campbell] has said, a fear among some clinicians about using three potentially hepatotoxic drugs, the actual rates of hepatotoxicity were 4 per cent in the non-pyrazinamide-containing regimen and 4 per cent in the pyrazinamide-containing regimens.

Darbyshire: I just thought I should carry on the story a little further, because that was Africa. But to me, that's where we should start from, because that's where it all started. But I think the story in the UK is that the BTA studies, together with the Singapore and East African studies, clearly demonstrated that probably the best regimen was isoniazid–rifampicin for six months with two months of pyrazinamide and a fourth drug. But I think the great debate in recent times in the UK is whether you actually need that fourth drug and here the dilemma is all to do with initial isoniazid resistance. So one of the questions which I think we have debated a number of times, and we have written guidelines about, is whether you need that initial fourth drug or not.[85] So that's another quite interesting route that we might like to go down. Then we could discuss Hong Kong and Singapore, and intermittent chemotherapy, if you like.

Girling: I think that is a very important point, because the key regimen that was actually recommended by the International Union Against Tuberculosis and Lung Disease was a three-drug regimen, rifampicin/isoniazid for six months with pyrazinamide for the first two, but they point out that that didn't have to be given daily, it could be given twice or three times a week; and they then went on to suggest some cheaper alternatives for developing countries.[86]

[84a] Dr Joseph Angel wrote: 'Incidentally, Figure 3 shows that the pyrazinamide-containing regimens produced more rapid sputum conversion than did the non-pyrazinamide-containing regimen.' Note on draft transcript, 20 July 2005.

[85] See, for example, Ormerod (2001); Joint Tuberculosis Committee of the British Thoracic Society (1998).

[86] International Union Against Tuberculosis and Lung Disease (1988).

Darbyshire: So even though we didn't call it DOTS [directly observed therapy short-course strategy], we were doing DOTS.[87]

Girling: Yes, and of course that raises the whole issue of intermittent administration as well.

Mitchison: That's not what DOTS is. DOTS is a five-point strategy, and has nothing to do with directly observed treatment, or with short-course treatment, either. It's now a complete misnomer you see, but it's a five-point strategy. It includes short-course chemotherapy and supervised treatment, but also government support, smear examinations for diagnosis, proper follow-ups, and proper drug supplies. It's a whole catalogue of things, so let's not use the term DOTS here.[88]

Girling: Thank you very much, Denny, we take your point.

Professor Peter Ormerod: As somebody who was treated with the old-style regimens in 1957 and has helped bring in newer short-course regimens in practice, in the streptomycin versus ethambutol debate, there's no comparison between my personal experience of three months of intramuscular streptomycin at the age of seven, and patients' joy at taking ethambutol, rather than streptomycin later. As somebody who had very little buttock at the age of seven, it was not a very pleasant experience, and sleeping on my front for three months was the result, though I am not deaf.

Citron: There is a study that we haven't mentioned, that seems to me is absolutely fundamental to our routine practice. And that is the 1959 study in Madras of home versus sanatorium treatment.[89] It showed that domiciliary

---

[87] World Health Organization (1994); Bayer and Wilkinson (1995). See also www.wellcome.ac.uk/doc_WTX024571.html (visited 11 May 2005). See also World Health Organization (1999).

[88] The DOTS (directly observed therapy short-course strategy) has been promoted by the WHO since the early 1990s. It consists of five elements: (i) government commitment to sustained tuberculosis-control activities; (ii) case detection by sputum-smear microscopy among symptomatic patients; (iii) standardized treatment regimens lasting at least six to eight months for all confirmed sputum-smear-positive cases, with directly observed treatment for the initial two months; (iv) a regular, uninterrupted supply of all essential antituberculous drugs; and (v) a standardized recording and reporting system that allows assessment of treatment results for each patient and of the tuberculosis-control programme overall. See World Health Organization (1999).

[89] Tuberculosis Chemotherapy Centre, Madras (1959); Fox (1962a): 413–7, 473–8; Dawson *et al.* (1966).

chemotherapy was as effective as in the sanatorium and caused no more disease among household contacts. It had a profound effect on our practice here, so that by the end of the 1960s most of the tuberculosis sanatoria and hospitals were either closed or were closing down. It seemed to me that this was absolutely fundamental. The physicians are now treating tuberculosis in outpatient departments in this country, and I think we ought to give credit to that Madras Study for the major effect on our clinical practice.

Dr Geoff Scott: I am quite interested by the transition from the treatment for 18 months to the treatment for six months. Clinical trials were going on and results were coming up and I was doing some treatment, although I wasn't involved in any trials, but gradually treatment courses shortened. I remembered there was a study that I think the MRC did, which was to ask people what treatments they did give and the replies weren't very consistent with anything which had been recommended. They tended to be longer, people tended to give more treatment than was necessary. I wondered if those around the room can tell us a bit about research into practice and how you made this transition?

Citron: I will deal with that subject in some detail in my talk about how chemotherapy regimens were introduced into routine clinical practice, because it's interesting to see the difference between what people say they do and what they actually do.

Ormerod: I will wait until Ken [Citron] does that, because last year I published the latest review of what treatment was actually given in 1998 in *Clinical Medicine*.[90] We have done follow-up studies, and the MRC in combination with the British Thoracic Society (BTS),[91] followed up what treatment was given in the surveys in 1983, 1988, 1993 and 1998.[92] I know it's not quite the past, but it showed what happens, and it does mirror how short-course chemotherapy was brought in. It was in 1988 that pyrazinamide-containing regimens were the rule rather than the exception, whereas in 1983 only about 11 per cent of people were on a pyrazinamide-containing regimen.

---

[90] Ormerod and Prescott (2003).

[91] The British Thoracic and Tuberculosis Association (BTTA) changed its name to the British Thoracic Association (BTA) in 1977, and to the British Thoracic Society (BTS) in 1982. See Snell (1978).

[92] British Thoracic Society (1984); Joint Tuberculosis Committee of the British Thoracic Society (1990, 1994, 1998).

Campbell: Again, going back to the first British Thoracic and Tuberculosis Association's (BTTA) trial that started in 1972. What impressed me, as a very junior research fellow helping to run this trial, was first of all the people of a very conservative nature, with a little 'c', that is the doctors, were going to go ahead with a new project, testing new ideas, and I think a lot of the credit for that must come from the earlier MRC study that was done in England and Wales, and the Scottish studies done by Sir John. The chest physicians, by this time, were a fairly disciplined bunch, accustomed to being led into doing studies. What became apparent during the trial, and this might give a context, was that senior physicians would ring this boy up in Edinburgh and ask him: is it really safe to stop these drugs now? What do you think I should do? And these were a number of very senior people ringing up. They had taken part, but their attitude was still, 'I am not terribly certain, can I give it for a little bit longer?' And I would say, 'No, you are not allowed, it's a clinical trial.' It is very salutary and I think it will have bearing on what Peter and Ken [Citron] are going to say later on, even after the results of the trial were published, people thinking, 'I will give it another two or three months', superstition influencing science.[93]

Crofton: Can I comment on what Ken [Citron] was talking about? In the first Madras study comparing sanatorium and home treatment, the patients at home in the slums were also intended to be on bed rest. But, of course, as they improved many of them no longer stayed in bed. Before that trial we had become so impressed with the success of chemotherapy that we thought that many of the milder, overtly noninfectious, patients might do adequately if they received chemotherapy while continuing to lead normal lives. We had a tremendous business trying to persuade the Scottish physicians that such a controlled trial was ethical because everybody thought that you needed at least three months' bed rest. We ran the study, they had the same chemotherapy, either for three months in bed, or living normal lives, and of course the ones living normal lives did just as well.[94]

Mitchison: Can I add one point to this? The person who started this was Philip D'Arcy Hart, because he organized the first clinical trial on streptomycin.[95] He had to deal with the fundamental conservatism of physicians. It's a great pity

---

[93] Monie *et al.* (1982).

[94] Tuberculosis Society of Scotland (1960).

[95] Medical Research Council (1948). See biographical note on page 102.

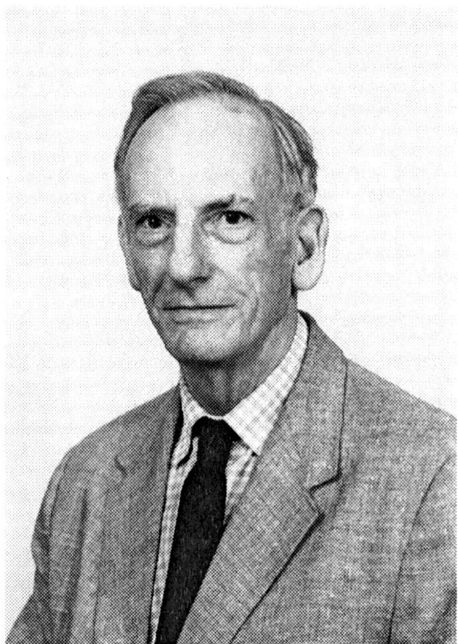

Figure 4: Dr Philip D'Arcy Hart in the 1950s.

he's not here, but he's still alive, and I think one ought to recognize the huge debt I believe we all owe to him, in getting clinical trials started. [Hear, hear.]

Jindani: Can I just say, in contrast, that my African colleagues, whenever they were presented with a trial that was going to be innovative, particularly six months, they were really excited about it, because if these came about, six-month trials, imagine how it would improve their practice and the possibility for eradicating tuberculosis. So I never encountered any resistance at all from my participants out there.

Crofton: I would like to draw attention to the identical problem in Russia, where they don't want to give up their old system and use the WHO regimen.[96] There's a very good example of how powerful conservatism can be.

Chalmers: I want to add a further plug for Philip D'Arcy Hart (Figure 4). On 22 June 2004, three days before Philip's 104th birthday, at the Royal College

[96] Hønneland and Rowe (2004): 49–56.

of Physicians, there will be a celebration of the sixtieth anniversary of the patulin trial. This is a much-underrated trial, which was beautifully done by Philip D'Arcy Hart, with the late Joan Faulkner, as she then was, being the driving force behind it.[97]

Campbell: Iain, what was the patulin trial?

Chalmers: It was the first properly controlled, multicentred trial done under the aegis of the MRC. Patulin was an antibiotic that Professor Harold Raistrick, from the London School of Hygiene and Tropical Medicine, felt was going to be useful in a number of ways. There were some case reports suggesting that it was good for the common cold and then there were a couple of small trials, one done in the navy by Surgeon Commander Hopkins, which suggested that it had an effect, and then other trials done in the army by Dr Stansfeld, which failed to replicate the findings in naval personnel. A large multicentred, very well controlled trial was done under the aegis of the MRC. Philip D'Arcy Hart was the principal driving force, and he was the secretary to the oversight committee. The assistant secretary was Joan (Faulkner, the late Lady Doll). It's a beautifully done trial and the whole paper will be reproduced, together with some historical papers and commentaries, and published in the April 2004 issue of the *International Journal of Epidemiology* to celebrate this sixtieth anniversary.[98]

Mitchison: Could I make the point here that the patulin trials didn't have a randomized intake? That was the one way in which they weren't quite the forerunner of modern clinical trials.

Chalmers: I think it's quite important to recognize there's no statistical advantage to random allocation over strict alternation.[99] The key thing is whether an unbiased allocation schedule is concealed successfully from those people who are entering patients. What is special about the patulin trial is that there were two identical drug groups, and two identical placebo groups. It is

---

[97] Medical Research Council, Patulin Clinical Trials Committee (1944); Clinical trials ran from December 1943 to April 1944, supervised by Dr Joan Faulkner. See also D'Arcy Hart (1999); Chalmers and Clarke (2004); Chalmers (2005).

[98] Chalmers and Clarke (2004).

[99] For details of Bradford Hill's first attempt to introduce the concept of randomization in controlled trials, see Wilkinson (1997). See also Yoshioka (1998); D'Arcy Hart (1999); Chalmers (2005).

clear from papers at the National Archive as well as from Philip D'Arcy Hart's memory, that they used these four groups to muddle people up, to ensure that it was less likely that they would vitiate the allocation schedule.[100] So it was a key study methodologically. Perhaps the reason that it has not received the attention that the streptomycin for pulmonary tuberculosis trial has is because of the magic reference to random sampling numbers in the report of the streptomycin trial, but not in the patulin trial. I think Philip D'Arcy Hart is right to say that the patulin trial was the first properly controlled multicentre trial done under the aegis of the MRC.[101]

Campbell: David, we are still, I think, on short-course regimens, aren't we? Others have voiced their 20-year questions. My 20-year question is directed to you and to Janet as disciples of Wallace, and to Sir John: we know that twice weekly therapy for the continuation phase is as efficient as daily, supplementing the first two months of an intensive phase. Why is that not recommended therapy in Britain?

Girling: The International Union recommendations did say that treatment could be given intermittently three times a week, or twice a week. That brings us on to the whole question of intermittency, which I think is another one that would be good for us to cover today on the suitability of some drugs and not others for intermittent use and the effectiveness of intermittent drug administration and its supervision. Of course, this is another area where there have been hugely important parallel developments of the clinical trials and the laboratory work. I think this was largely Jean Dickinson's work on the guinea-pig experiments. Perhaps, Denny, you could start by telling us a bit about these, because these were really quite important findings, weren't they? They were, to some extent, quite unexpected as to what might happen if you gave certain antituberculosis drugs once a week or every day? She studied different intervals, didn't she, between drug administrations?

Mitchison: What she was mainly concerned with, in the *in vitro*, in the test-tube experiments, was simply giving the bacilli a pulse of drug lasting various times from two up to 96 hours. From those it became evident that if you

---

[100] Chalmers and Clarke (2004).

[101] Medical Research Council, Patulin Clinical Trials Committee (1944); Medical Research Council (1948); Landsborough (1975): 238–9; Chalmers and Clarke (2004).

pulsed with isoniazid, first of all the pulses were cumulative, a fact of great importance, because a lot of small pulses add up to give a maximal lag that lasted about seven to eight days. This agreed well with what happened in the intermittent isoniazid/streptomycin trials in Madras, where when you gave the drugs twice weekly, so you got fairly frequent pulses, the slow and the rapid inactivators behaved the same. But when you got to once weekly treatment, the small pulse in the rapid inactivators didn't last until the next pulse, whereas the big pulse in the slows did. So that was the basis to explain that particular set of effects. Also it was the opposite of what happened with rifampicin which has an immediate bactericidal effect, followed by a gradual recovery with an almost immediate start. Now, this has a bearing on things happening at the moment, particularly in the use of once weekly rifapentine in HIV-positive patients, and the emergence of monoresistance to rifamycins, because there's a gap in the effect of rifapentine, which there isn't in the effect of isoniazid.[102] These postantibiotic effects were explored for the then current drugs, all of which have slightly different characteristics. That work has not, as far as I know, been extended in any meaningful way.

Campbell: Was it not the Singapore study, David [Girling], that showed you could give intensive therapy for two months, and then rifampicin and isoniazid for four months twice a week and get the same results as daily? [Yes.] I am intrigued that that has not crept into routine practice, and I am not talking about supervision now, I am asking why has it not crept in? Why are we still stuck with daily? How did this not arise as it were, or not happen?

Girling: I think it is routine practice, as I understand it, in Singapore, and in Hong Kong now. Well, during the trials in Hong Kong, they got used to the idea of organizing their entire treatment service on a three-times weekly basis and patients came Mondays, Wednesdays and Fridays, or Tuesdays, Thursdays, and Saturdays, and it was so well organized that they were in and out of the clinic, just like that; their drugs were waiting for them. We talked a little time ago about the communist regimes. In Prague, for example, in Czechoslovakia, considerable success was achieved by enabling treatment to be supervised at various different places. People could have their treatment supervised at their

---

[102] Rifapentine is a rifamycin (see note 34) with a long half-life. Studies *in vitro* and in experimental murine tuberculosis suggest that it would be effective if given once weekly. See Dickinson and Mitchison (1987); Mitchison *et al.* (1988). See also Sirgel *et al.* (2005).

place of work, for example.[103] So I think in some countries it has caught on, and not in others. I am not sure about Czechoslovakia now.

Mitchison: Could I make a point that in the USA if you say that you want daily continuation therapy, they say it's impossible, they will only give intermittent chemotherapy, so quite clearly there are totally different ideas in different countries?

Darbyshire: I was just going to say that I think one of the issues here is whether it is supervised or not, because I think the great danger of moving over into intermittent treatment that's not supervised, will be that it is much less likely to be taken properly. I think people find it much harder to take something twice a week than they do daily, and therefore we in this country are focused on daily treatment, because we have relatively little supervised treatment. I think it's a practical thing.

Citron: Could I ask Peter Ormerod about the surveys that the BTS has done? In a situation which is predominantly daily, self-administered chemotherapy regimens, are we getting very good results? I can say that intermittency is used a fair amount at this time. My own practice with the homeless and alcoholics and so on, and I think John Moore-Gillon will bear this out, that those people who are likely to be unreliable need supervised therapy and get twice weekly or three-times weekly therapy in their own hostels, or in hospitals, or in the places they go to have meals and so on. It is certainly used selectively.

Ormerod: In the BTS guidance, it is allowed to give intermittent treatment, in fact thrice weekly is the recommended regimen for people who are thought likely to be noncompliant, but the drug dosages also include a twice weekly dosing option. The surveys that we have done following up the 1998 and 1993 surveys show that we are getting reasonably good results with daily treatment, which is the norm but not the rule: with cure and completion rates of over 80 per cent in those people who return the forms, and it's as good as any comparison with cohort studies across Europe. But there isn't always compliance monitoring, people are not using the four-drug initial

---

[103] Dr David Girling wrote: 'The organization of fully supervised chemotherapy must be efficient and flexible so that patients can choose to receive their chemotherapy at centres near their home, near, at, or on the way to their place of work, or at some other place convenient for them. Such centres can include chest clinics, general practitioners' surgeries, dispensaries, welfare clinics, hospitals, factory clinics, rural health units and special treatment stations, such as can be set up on market days in rural areas. See Fox (1979).' Letter to Dr Daphne Christie, 8 April 2005.

combination in ethnic groups with isoniazid resistance rates of 7 per cent, these ethnic groups now making up over 70 per cent of all cases in the UK, and there is a risk of failure from that. With reference to Denny's comment about the availability of anything other than twice weekly continuation therapy in the USA: in the USA it is mainly three times weekly if given intermittently. But when you do studies, the Americans say they are giving DOTS. When they did a national analysis three years ago, only 15 per cent were actually getting supervised treatment, not anything like the numbers that they say they are. It should come with a health warning, some of their statistics.

Girling: Amina, do you have any feel, internationally, of the extent to which intermittency is being used and, of course, full supervision or not?

Jindani: That was the point I was going to make, that at the moment I am coordinating international multicentre trials in Latin America, Asia and Africa. Most of the Latin American and Asian countries give intermittent therapy in the continuation phase, which they claim is fully supervised, with good results.

Crofton: Can I come in briefly on this? Denny and I were both at the WHO meeting which made this formal recommendation, but there was a good deal of discussion as to whether it should be twice a week or three times a week. The general feeling was that they were nervous about reducing it to twice a week, and the recommendation was three times a week. The basis of this decision, I think, depended quite a lot on the Singapore study.

Angel: It has been claimed by some streptomycin defenders, that if you keep streptomycin for these fractious patients on whom you wish to use twice- or three-times weekly treatment, this is an advantage. Would anybody like to say anything about that?

Girling: What, because it encourages compliance; because they need injections, do you mean?

Campbell: Betraying my ignorance again: Janet [Darbyshire] said that patients prefer to take tablets daily. I would like to ask Janet, if there is any evidence of that from studies, even of surveys asking patients which they would prefer, twice weekly or a daily tablet? I don't know of any myself, but I am a very ignorant person.

Darbyshire: I think it has been confirmed that people will not remember. What I was saying was not so much that the patients might prefer it, but the concern is that it is actually much more difficult to remember to take something twice a week, so there's the worry about compliance, not that it's the patient that prefers it. I don't know if any studies have tested that, except that at one time we went a long way down planning one – although we actually had placebo on the other days, because we were very worried that people wouldn't take it the other days. So it may be that the book by Sackett,[104] which was one of Wallace's favourites on compliance, has a study, I know we looked at how to give intermittent nonsupervised treatment, and as I say we got a long way down developing a packet that had two days of active within a week of pills that all looked the same. I will go back and look at Sackett and let you know if it's there.

Campbell: It will be very difficult to have a placebo that doesn't contain rifampicin – the patients will know which days they are taking their active treatment, because they would have orange urine.

Darbyshire: That's maybe why we didn't do it.

Jindani: On this point about recommended short-course regimens: it's become evident to me that the different countries in the world use different short-course regimens, and the Republic of Guinea, in spite of their rising prevalence of HIV, still give streptomycin as an inducement to make the patient come daily for the first two months of treatment. There are other countries like that.

Dr Bertie Squire: I am very much a newcomer to the scene, but very interested in this question of intermittency. Henry Mwandumba from Malawi and I were interested in whether intermittency was possible from much earlier in short-course regimens, and are responsible for the Cochrane Systematic Review, which pulled out evidence for head-to-head comparisons of intermittency versus daily dosing right from the second week onwards. If we have got it right, and we did try very hard, there is only one comparison that is two parts of one of the Hong Kong trials, which actually compares intermittent dosing from very early on. I just wanted to add that into the debate, because I think what I have been hearing is a debate about intermittency during the continuation phase. But it often gets spread into a question about intermittency from much earlier on, which is of huge programme importance, if you are trying to organize direct supervision on a community basis, in African situations.

Davies: I recall being interviewed by Wallace Fox for an MRC job in the middle of the summer of 1978. It was a fascinating experience. I got more and more transfixed by the fact that Wallace was never able to take a sip of coffee,

---

[104] Sackett and Snow (1979): 11–22. See also Mitchison (1998).

because he was always asking questions, or listening to answers. But one thing he asked me, I remember, was what regimen did my bosses use? At that time I had been working as a senior house officer and registrar in west London, and, of course, none of my bosses used anything like the regimens that were by then being recommended at the MRC. It was a source of Wallace's frustration that he couldn't get his message across to the ordinary punter, to the chest physician in the street, and this led Wallace in the early 1980s to write a couple of papers, I recall, on the lack of compliance by chest physicians in fulfilling the MRC criteria that he had worked out so thoroughly.[105] Janet [Darbyshire] mentioned the fact that we give daily therapy, because patients can take it at home. We observe intermittent regimens because that's the way that we can make sure that the patients take the medication. But I would like to throw another question in here, and that is the one about side-effects. Like Ian Campbell, who trained me in tuberculosis, to some extent I share his ignorance: I cannot recall whether adverse effects were an issue in using intermittent as opposed to daily regimens, but I guess they must have been.

Girling: We will come to adverse effects after tea.

Mitchison: Can I say something about the history of this? It arose immediately after the Madras home sanatorium comparison, and it was quite evident to Wallace, and indeed to all of us, that we had to do something about compliance. You see we were throwing chemotherapy open to the world, we had to do something. The first step was to look at supervised intermittent chemotherapy. Most of the important studies then were done at Madras. So, if one wants to go back historically, one has to go back to Madras. It was only later that the possibility of shortened treatment came up as an even more effective way of ensuring compliance. And toxicity came into it very early on. Wallace's slides that he showed always had the statement that intermittent treatment reduces toxicity.

Moore-Gillon: I was going to ask a question. Coming back to something that Sir John [Crofton] said about the meeting at the WHO, and then Peter Davies mentioned the same sort of problem. Presumably the issuing of guidelines is partly the art of the possible, not just the evidence that you have got in front of you, because having persuaded one's colleagues that they didn't need to treat for 18 months, but only for a short period of time, that's quite a big jump to take on board. To then say, 'Well, you only need it twice a week as well', was an even bigger step to take, but you thought you might be able to swing three

---

[105] Fox (1983a, 1983b).

times a week past them. Was there some judgement made as to what was going to be possible to persuade people to do in making these recommendations?

Crofton: Denny may remember the discussion, but I cannot remember it very clearly, but there was obviously nervousness about the twice a week. Do you remember what the worry was?

Mitchison: The issue was that if you forgot one of your twice weekly doses, then you would have a once weekly treatment which had been shown not to work very well. So I think it was the nervousness about what would happen with the missed doses that pushed people towards three times a week.

Crofton: I think I ought to point out that one of the reasons why we got such good results in Edinburgh was that we always tested the urine for drugs at every attendance so we knew when people weren't taking their drugs. We always kept it quiet, and in my entire career I had only two patients who realized what was happening, that they were being tested, because we never said, 'Oh your urine is negative'. We said, 'I'm not sure things are going so well, you'd better be admitted for a little bit'. Or, 'You must be very careful to take all your drugs every day' and then bring them back to the clinic shortly to retest their urine, if necessary readmitting them to ensure they completed treatment.

Girling: Before we break for tea in about eight minutes' time, we have said nothing as yet about the management of extrapulmonary tuberculosis.[106] The original International Union Recommendations recommended short-course chemotherapy for both pulmonary and extrapulmonary disease. So does anyone have anything they would like to share with us on the management of extrapulmonary disease? Ian, I think you were involved in the lymph node trials, is that right?

Campbell: Yes, because again when I was a BTTA research fellow on Sir John's unit, the Clinical Trials Subcommittee of the Research Committee came up with a idea of doing short-course chemotherapy in lymph node tuberculosis, which raised a huge fuss, because everybody thought lymph node tuberculosis was a grim disease that never really went away and usually came back. When you look at the literature, as that group did – Elizabeth Hills will remember this – what had been done previously in lymph node tuberculosis was inadequate or just anecdotal. When we did that first trial, 18 months was included as a sort of sop to Reg Bignall: 'Let's keep this 18 months in, chaps, and we will go for the nine as well, and the 12'. That was much more challenging than doing the

[106] Dr David Girling wrote: 'The MRC spinal tuberculosis trials and other aspects of extrapulmonary tuberculosis are summarized in Girling *et al.* (1988).' Letter to Dr Daphne Christie, 28 July 2004.

short-course trial for pulmonary. The first short-course trial for lymph node tuberculosis, done by the BTTA, was the first-ever randomized, controlled clinical trial of lymph node tuberculosis.[107] It also served as the first prospective survey of that disease under treatment. So it was a very interesting study, but it raised everybody's fears because the disease was dreaded so much.

Girling: They weren't still using the Queen's touch, I suppose?

Campbell: Yes, perhaps some people were! The present Queen was on the throne by then, wasn't she? Yes. But some people not too far away on your right[108] still think that sunlight and vitamin D might help this disease, you know.

Girling: Would anybody else like to comment on extrapulmonary tuberculosis?

Glynn: These are two completely anecdotal, probably not very useful, but rather amusing, stories. First from St Mary's: in the 1950s, there was a trial on treatment of tuberculous meningitis. I went there just after that trial had finished, so I was never involved in it, but we still used to get patients with tuberculous meningitis referred. They were treated with streptomycin, among other things, sometimes intrathecally.[109] At some stage one of them developed a block and it became impossible to give him streptomycin by lumbar puncture. We thought we might have some burr holes [little holes in the skull, made by a burr drill] and he was referred to Mr Dickson-Wright,[110] who said, 'Rubbish, get on with it'. He was referred again with some pressure by Professor Neuberger, and I came in one morning at about 9.00am and was told to go to Dickson-Wright in theatre immediately. I was then the senior registrar. I got there and Dickie was doing some major operation, I don't know what, with his mask hanging well below his nose, and he said, 'Well, this is how you need to give this, by cisternal puncture, this is how you would do it,' and

---

107 Campbell and Dyson (1977).

108 Dr John Moore-Gillon wrote: 'This was a humorous reference to Peter Davies.' Note on draft transcript, 25 April 2005. Dr Ian Campbell wrote: 'I was indicating that at the time of the study referred to earlier, the present Queen was already on the throne, and might have been approached by old-fashioned patients/physicians to touch the patient and thereby cure their disease (scrofula = extrapulmonary TB = lymph node TB). David Girling was referring to the Middle Ages when some believed that the Royal touch would cure that disease. I was being jocular.' Edited from a letter to Dr Daphne Christie, 7 June 2005.

109 Cairns *et al.* (1946).

110 Professor Alan Glynn wrote: 'A consultant surgeon at St Mary's Hospital, famous for his irascibility.' E-mail to Dr Daphne Christie, 8 April 2005.

explained how to do a cisternal puncture in about two minutes flat, and said, 'Go away and do it'. So I did. Much to my surprise, the patient survived and actually got better. I was terrified at one end of the needle, I don't think he [the patient] was surprised at the other, because he didn't know what was happening.

The other story was at St Mary's too. At that time there was a relic of a so-called boils clinic among other things. One day a lady of about 50 or so came up, a school teacher, who many years before had tuberculosis glands in the neck, for which she had been treated by the people there at that time with injections of something called 'tubercle powder'. I looked at the notes, which were really a history of injections, week after week, or month after month, and that was all. The nurse, or the amateur nurse actually, I think, she was, gave me a bottle of tubercle powder, it said on the label it was that, and said you give her this. I thought, no way can I give her this. This bottle is ancient, the rubber top was so dry it was cracked and there was a sort of nasty stuff inside.[111] So I tried to persuade her not to have it, that she was better now, but she said no I must have it. So I gave her an injection of saline. She never came back; I don't know whether she died.

Girling: Thank you for those historical insights.

Darbyshire: I thought I should mention what took up quite a lot of my life at one time, namely the tuberculosis spine studies, which again were a series of studies, the first set used standard treatment and looked at different ways of managing the disease, and which showed that bed rest was of no benefit, plaster jackets were of no benefit and debridement was of no benefit.[112] This was a programme in Korea, Hong Kong, Bulawayo and South Africa. But the second set of studies did look at short-course chemotherapy, again in Hong Kong and Korea, and also in Madras this time, and showed that just six months of rifampicin plus isoniazid – I don't know quite why we didn't put pyrazinamide in, but maybe Denny [Mitchison] will tell me why we didn't – was actually very highly effective. The only benefit was from this radical surgery in Hong Kong where they developed the technique, but the benefits were really quite small. So I think those series of studies really defined the management of spinal tuberculosis and the role of short-course chemotherapy.

---

[111] Professor Alan Glynn thinks that the tubercle powder was most probably derived from tubercle bacilli.

[112] See, for example, Medical Research Council Working Party on Tuberculosis of the Spine (1976, 1978, 1999).

Sir Christopher Booth: Can we go back to tuberculous meningitis? Because that was an appalling condition, and treating small children with intrathecal injections was a disastrous experience for all doctors who had to deal with it. My understanding is that there were some very good trials in South Africa and elsewhere in Africa that produced regimens there. Could somebody comment on what those regimens were and how it happened?

Girling: I have to say I am not familiar with those trials. Does anyone else know about them?

Mitchison: I do know a little bit about them, but they have been mainly done by Peter Donald at the University of Stellenbosch, near Cape Town, because he is very much a paediatric specialist, although he's done a lot with adult tuberculosis. I have been on his ward rounds where half of his patients tend to have miliary or tuberculous meningitis. It's quite phenomenal how much there is. He's done a long series [of studies] treated with six months of isoniazid and rifampicin.[113] What I think is quite evident about tuberculous meningitis, and about bone and joint tuberculosis, is that you don't have the same problem about drug resistance, because your bacterial populations are much smaller, so you are concerned with just killing the bugs, not with preventing drug resistance. As rifampicin is the most important drug for shortening treatment, it's a key drug in this combination. But, of course, isoniazid penetrates very well into the lesions.

Ormerod: I will expand on what Ian Campbell said. The BTS have done a further study, which he chaired, looking at six months versus nine months, so we have actually shown with six months' regimens that they are just as effective for lymph node tuberculosis.

One final comment about South Africa. I think they use ethionamide there sometimes as a fourth drug, rather than ethambutol, because of better penetration of the CSF [cerebro-spinal fluid].

Citron: I don't think we ought to forget the studies done by Sister Mary Aquinas and Sister M Gabriel in Hong Kong on tuberculous meningitis.[114] Again, they confirmed the value of ethionamide and pyrazinamide, which I

---

[113] See Donald *et al.* (1998).

[114] Aquinas (1974).

believe penetrates very well into the CSF, and of course rifampicin and isoniazid. She did a series of studies over almost a decade with extremely good results, except in the advanced cases.[115] Essentially, the prognosis depends on the stage at which the patients present with this disease. In stages 1 and 2 she got extremely good results.

Crofton: Perhaps after tea somebody could say something about using steroids in these diseases like meningitis.

Girling: Gaye Fox is now going to say a few words about her experiences in Madras, I think, with Wallace.

Mrs Gaye Fox: I am very pleased to attend the seminar, but I am awfully sad that Wallace cannot be here himself.[116] Wallace went to Madras, as you probably all know, in 1956, when he embarked on his famous studies, which led to short-course chemotherapy. I remember him telling me one day that somebody's got to do a study on home versus sanatorium, so I am sticking my neck out! From that study came the contact study, and I think, Janet [Darbyshire], from that there was a compliance study. From that followed the shorter and shorter courses of chemotherapy, and I really wonder if there were ever any more important studies than those undertaken in the Madras centre. These were done in very difficult conditions. It was said that the Indians might not be cooperative, but with a dedicated team the patients were persuaded to cooperate and the studies had very few absconders. The climate was also notoriously hostile, and yet many of the staff worked long hours, and Wallace usually worked an 18-hour day, often bringing colleagues back to chew over the problems in the evening. There was no air conditioning at all for the first two years, no machines for sorting out statistical cards, hence the statistical cards were sorted out by hand, in their thousands without even the benefits of a fan to cool the room. Fans would have blown the cards about!

Wallace also had something to contend with that I think you would have all dreaded, he had to answer to four separate bodies: the Madras Government, the Indian Government, the WHO and the MRC. How many of you would enjoy that prospect! Sometimes they didn't always understand the problems in the field.

---

[115] See, for example, Humphries *et al.* (1990).

[116] Two tributes to Wallace Fox are given in Appendix 1. Sent from Mrs Wallace Fox to Dr Daphne Christie, 19 March 2005. See also biographical note on page 101.

When he finally returned to the UK he was occupied with studies all over the world, and where he used his usual creative ability, designing studies to suit all the varied conditions. For example, the Bedouins in Algeria, overcrowding in Hong Kong, communist Czechoslovakia; each one was designed to make the best use of the best way to look after the patients to ensure they took their drugs. And just to sum up, because Wallace cannot talk for himself, I hope that you, his colleagues and friends, will strive to ensure that the work he pioneered in Madras and later, that was undertaken all over the world is not forgotten and his name is not buried in history.

Girling: Thank you very much indeed. Now we are going to have a session on the role of steroids in the management of tuberculosis. Now John, you brought this up. Do you want to say a few words to introduce it?

Crofton: We did a study in Scotland on pulmonary tuberculosis and it was a controlled trial, and they were randomized, all having standard chemotherapy and in one group, 20 mg prednisolone a day, if I remember, for three months, and the other no steroids. They were assessed at the end, and the initial results were quite dramatic. The patients' X-rays cleared more quickly, they felt much better more quickly, and they gained weight more quickly. No effect on sputum at all. We then did a follow-up a year later to try to compare the two groups, because we thought that the prednisone might have decreased fibrosis in the lungs. So we did blind readings of the X-rays and we couldn't find any fibrosis that had not already been present at the beginning, as far as you could judge from the X-ray. So, it made no difference long term, but there was some immediate effect.[117] One of the reasons we did this was that there had been a lot of controversy in the medical press. Some doctors had given corticosteroids to counter allergic reactions to the drugs and had been impressed by dramatic improvement both subjectively and radiologically. Then other places said they had used it, and it was absolutely disastrous. Reading the literature rather carefully, I thought the ones that had gone wrong were those who were giving bad chemotherapy and getting resistance. So we thought that it was justifiable to do a trial of this kind. The BTTA did a later trial, but unfortunately they didn't do a year's assessment; they found the same things in the early stages, but they didn't do a blind reading after a year to see whether it affected the

---

[117] Horne (1960).

X-ray. Then, of course, other people tried it. I don't think the MRC did a trial in meningitis, but they did one in pericarditis in South Africa.[118]

There's been a lot of controversy over the years about how useful steroids would be in meningitis, but there was a controlled trial done in India, actually on pleural effusion, which was a reasonably good one and it did show the effect. I don't know of any controlled trial on meningitis. For years we have had so little. But the conclusion seemed to be in recent years, when we were doing our book, that it seemed to be established that it was useful, but somebody here can perhaps tell us about it more scientifically.

Mitchison: I think I should add that there was a very big and rather important study in pulmonary tuberculosis, well controlled with follow-ups that showed no effect of steroids at all.[119] Now, I have heard from Guy Thwaites who claims to have got a very definite answer from a very big study of tuberculous meningitis in Vietnam. This is quite recently, and he says that he has incontrovertible evidence that it does have a positive beneficial effect. But this is not yet published as far as I know. It was used at the beginning of treatment of pulmonary tuberculosis in Madras, in high dosage. It was randomized. It was a factorial study with two treatments.[120]

Crofton: Were you looking at X-rays and patients and weights and things?

Mitchison: The whole lot, probably even more than in Edinburgh, because it was done at a rather later date.

Crofton: Yes, but ours wasn't an Edinburgh study, it was a Scottish study.

Mitchison: Oh, Scottish study, I beg your pardon. But I think this issue has been settled with regard to pulmonary tuberculosis, both in a non-short-course trial, which is yours, and in a short-course trial, which is the Madras one.

Crofton: Yes, I don't think there's any particular point in patients who are not very ill, but I was fairly convinced to begin with that we had several patients who came in moribund, and these would often die and they often had electrolyte upsets. We felt that by giving steroids they improved fairly quickly and we kept them alive for the chemotherapy to take effect.

---

[118] Steroids are anti-inflammatory drugs and thought to reduce the accumulation of pericardial fluid or prevent the development of adhesions in the pericardium which are induced by the tuberculous infection. See Strang *et al.* (1987, 1988); Ntsekhe *et al.* (2003).

[119] Tuberculosis Research Centre, Madras (1983).

[120] Thwaites *et al.* (2004).

Mitchison: I remember that effect in your report, but it didn't turn up again in the Madras study I am pretty sure, because we were well aware of that report, you see, at the time and I think there was a completely negative result in Madras.

Crofton: I wonder why?

Angel: I did a study of adrenocorticotropic hormone (ACTH) rather than prednisone when I was in the USA. I corroborate what Professor Crofton says about moribund patients, they certainly were saved. The other point was that the X-ray changes were quite remarkable, that somebody with very extensive tuberculosis radiographically cleared up within a couple of months. We gave the ACTH for three months and then withdrew it gradually and, of course, you got a rebound on the X-ray, it sort of clouded up again. Unfortunately at that time we didn't, I didn't, appreciate the absolute importance of bacteriology, and the follow-up was rather short, because I came back to the UK.

Mitchison: Was this a comparative trial?

Angel: Yes it was streptomycin, PAS and isoniazid for six months, with or without ACTH.

Nunn: I thought I would say a few words about the pericarditis study in Transkei in South Africa. It was a remarkable study in several respects. First of all when George Strang came to the MRC's Tuberculosis and Chest Diseases Unit and told us about these cases of tuberculous pericarditis, nobody believed the extent of the problem. In fact, over 350 patients were enrolled in that study from one hospital in the Transkei – a study funded by the Wellcome Trust, incidentally. Patients were randomized to prednisolone or placebo for three weeks, in addition to the standard short-course chemotherapy. The results were impressive in terms of reducing the need for further pericardiocentesis, or pericardiectomy, and survival rates improved. We have recently been writing up the ten-year follow-up for that study, over 95 per cent of patients were followed and there's a significant benefit in terms of mortality to those who were on the steroids compared with the placebo group.[121]

Citron: A question to Sir John. I think that Norman Horne produced some evidence that steroids were useful in renal tuberculosis, in preventing stricture of the ureter, so I would like to know what the evidence for that was?[122] May I

---

[121] Professor Andrew Nunn wrote: 'For the ten-year results see Strang *et al.* (2004).' Note on draft transcript, 28 July 2004.

[122] Horne and Tulloch (1975).

say that Sister Mary Aquinas, with her vast experience of tuberculous meningitis, was convinced that steroids should be given in stage 3 and in stage 2, and were particularly valuable for preventing CSF block. But I don't think she did a randomized study.

Mitchison: Can I make the point that the possibility of steroids making a difference to the results of chemotherapy, that is to say on the bacterial population, was investigated pretty thoroughly, both at Cornell by Walsh McDermott's group, and also by John Batten when he came back from New York. These experiments as well as his own showed quite clearly that steroid administration to murine tuberculosis makes absolutely no difference to the killing action of drugs.[123] But, of course, the thing that they could, and probably do, make a difference to is inflammation. I think one has to separate these two components.

Dr Freda Festenstein: I certainly recall in our clinical practice that in cases of severe drug reactions we used prednisolone and it was very effective indeed.

Crofton: As far as I can remember, Norman really did this by looking at what had happened in the people who were treated. I don't think there was a controlled trial; I don't think we had enough patients.

Dr Adrian Martineau: Just a comment. Is it possible that steroids are effective in very severe tuberculosis because these patients are Addisonian – they have adrenal tuberculosis?

Angel: If they were Addisonian they wouldn't respond to ACTH, would they? My study was with ACTH.

Dr Jeanette Meadway: I am very interested in all the discussion that I am listening to, because I am thinking how this points to the future, with more and more tuberculosis going to be something that's associated with HIV, more and more we will be thinking of treatment of the two conditions together. One thing that's very striking about patients with HIV who get tuberculosis is the proportion who have it with almost no localizing reaction, and you get something like a positive blood culture for *Mycobacterium tuberculosis* or a positive stool culture for *Mycobacterium tuberculosis* as the main sign, apart from the patient being nonspecifically unwell, maybe to the point of dying of the disease. But there's no localization. If patients start on antiretrovirals for

---

[123] Batten (1968); McCune *et al.* (1966).

their HIV, they then raise their CD4 count and start to get localizing symptoms, and this can be very severe. They get immune reconstitution syndrome (IRS) where they actually have a systemic upset that can be quite striking, or the localization can produce local symptoms which are major, such as a tuberculoma, which can suddenly precipitate raised intracranial pressure. The treatment for IRS is steroids. So maybe, if we look to the future – patients with HIV and tuberculosis – an extra question as well as which do you start first out of tuberculosis drugs and antiretrovirals, which antiretrovirals? Which tuberculosis drugs? There's another question there, which is whether you actually give steroids, thinking about the possibility of IRS?

Nunn: Just one quick comment. In a study, which was reported last year from Uganda, Alison Elliot assessed the role of prednisolone on HIV-infected patients with tuberculous pleural effusion, and found no benefit.

Girling: There was a Zimbabwe study wasn't there? Was that the one you were talking about?

Nunn: No, these were pleural effusions.

Girling: Yes, the Zimbabwe study was in pericarditis. But all their patients were HIV positive and they also found the benefit of steroids.[124] I think we probably ought to move on. The next topic is directly observed therapy. I think we have probably covered most of that unless anyone else has still got something that they are burning to say about supervision, or about directly observed therapy. How about you, Knut, have you got anything you would like to add on that to supervision of chemotherapy or directly observed therapy?

Dr Knut Øvreberg: As a matter of fact, directly observed therapy is the headline of the programme that is implemented by WHO and the IUATLD. But if you look at the results of therapy itself, there is good directly observed therapy, and there is directly observed therapy that is not so good. When I go, for example, to Nepal and observe the way the type of treatment is given, some patients come and take the drugs, but are not observed while they are taking the drugs, and therefore it is quite easy for patients to come, appear, take the drugs and throw them away. So directly observed therapy has to be really directly observed. If it's not directly observed, then it means that it doesn't comply with the principles that we know we are looking at.

---

[124] Hakim *et al.* (2000).

Davies: The point that needs to be made at the beginning of directly observed therapy is that it is only a means to an end, it is not an end in itself. The end in itself is twofold: one, if you are a public health doctor, to prevent the emergence of drug resistance; and two, if you are a clinician, to cure your patient. If you have in a community, in a service, cure rates of 85 per cent or better, and no emergence of drug resistance, then whatever method you are using, that's appropriate. But if you are not achieving that, then DOT is what you should be considering.

Moore-Gillon: This Witness Seminar is covering a period when people could be more creative in their choice of titles for their scientific journal papers, because there's a paper in the *Journal of the American Medical Association* from the 1960s entitled 'It's the skid row hotel manager who sees that Ernie takes his tuberculosis drugs' – that's the title of the paper.[125]

Jindani: I keep hearing that directly observed therapy was the invention of the WHO and the IUATLD, and I would like to correct that. There are two people we miss here greatly, one of course is Wallace Fox, and the other is Dr Pierce Kent, who was the Director of the East African Tuberculosis Investigation Centre in Nairobi,[126] and I had the great privilege of working for him. He invented directly observed therapy, particularly for patients with drug-resistant tuberculosis, on the basis that we had very few second-line drugs, and this constituted their last chance for survival. So that was an invention of Pierce Kent.

Darbyshire: I would just like to add a Pierce Kent story. One of the things I remember when I was very young is Pierce saying that he could solve tuberculosis if he had a blood test that you could use with a thumb prick, and an injection that you could give a month's treatment in people's bottoms.

Girling: Shall we move on to adverse effects of short-course regimens?[127] Now I think it's worth emphasizing yet again the importance of randomized clinical

---

[125] Fagerhaugh and Frankel (1970).

[126] Dr Amina Jindani wrote: 'This was an East African Community Research Centre which collaborated with the MRC in carrying out prevalence surveys as well as clinical trials in Kenya, Tanzania and Uganda. It was disbanded in 1979.' Note on draft transcript, 23 March 2005.

[127] Dr David Girling wrote: 'For a general account of adverse effects, see Girling (1982); also published in *Bulletin of the International Union Against Tuberculosis* 1984; **59**: 152–62. For a more detailed discussion of the hepatic toxicity of short-course chemotherapy see Girling (1978).' Letter to Dr Daphne Christie, 28 July 2004.

trials, and also indeed of the complementary laboratory research, because in this whole programme of trials there were large numbers of patients being studied in reliable, concurrent comparisons. Their treatment was being fully supervised, and so it's most unlikely that adverse effects were going to be missed. This programme also meant that we knew exactly how much of their drug patients had taken, how much they had actually received. It also enabled us to assemble data from many types of patient being studied in a large number of trials, and to study both single drugs and drug combinations. Reliable information was therefore obtained on the clinical characteristics of the adverse effects, their severity, their frequency, the effects of dose size and of the interval between doses and also on ways of managing them. Complementary laboratory research was invaluable in showing the mechanisms of some of these adverse effects, and also suggesting ways not only of treating them, but also of preventing them.

So I thought I would give one example to set us off on this session of adverse effects, and that's the example of the flu syndrome, an adverse effect of rifampicin when given intermittently.[128] A lot of information from the MRC trials showed that it occurred during intermittent [treatment], but very, very rarely during daily, administration. The clinical symptoms were fever, chills, malaise and headache. They appeared about three months after the start of treatment, and they started about one or two hours after a dose, and lasted for about eight hours. And of particular interest, their frequency varied with the dose, and also with the interval between doses of rifampicin, being more common with larger doses and, interestingly enough, with longer intervals between doses. So as you moved from twice weekly to once weekly, you got an increase in the incidence of the flu syndrome. It therefore became possible with this information to study, and indeed determine, drug doses of intermittently administered rifampicin that were both highly effective and associated with very low risk of reaction. In fact, episodes of the flu syndrome are now very rarely seen, or so I have been told, with the current intermittent doses recommended by the International Union.[129] Interestingly enough, episodes of the flu syndrome could be stopped by giving rifampicin daily instead of intermittently, even though the total dose was larger. Complementary laboratory research showed that it was associated with circulating rifampicin-

[128] Dr David Girling wrote: 'For a review of adverse effects of rifampicin, see Girling (1977).' Letter to Dr Daphne Christie, 28 July 2004.

[129] International Union Against Tuberculosis and Lung Disease (1988).

dependent antibodies; strongly suggesting it had an immunological nature. Indeed, research by Sister Gabriel in Hong Kong showed that the concentration of antibodies fell during an episode.[130] So it seems that rifampicin–antibody complexes were being formed, and the activation of complement was suggested as a possible mechanism. That's all I am going to say by way of introduction, but if people want to ask questions, or make other comments on adverse effects to the drugs, particularly those used in modern short-course chemotherapy, but not necessarily limited to those, please feel free to do so.

Citron: This information is, of course, very important to clinicians who are using daily rifampicin, because from time to time you see flu syndrome or, even worse, renal complications, in a patient who is supposed to be taking their rifampicin daily, but in fact is only taking it once or twice a week, or just when they turn up for the clinic. So it's very important to know about that.

Crofton: This is just a rather comic interlude. When isoniazid came in people were terribly impressed with what it did to the patients, they felt absolutely marvellous and it was thought that it might have a major metabolic effect on people, and some people said they felt wonderful. We did a controlled trial on ourselves, we did a double-blind switchover trial, and we were weighed every day with our backs to the scales, so that we couldn't see what was happening, and we recorded bad dreams and that sort of thing.[131] And of course it showed that nothing happened at all. But it was quite amusing the sort of symptoms that some people reported when they were on placebo: 'Never felt so wonderful', 'glorious dreams', and so on.

Girling: Somebody ought to do a study of the adverse effects of placebo.

Mitchison: Pyrazinamide, now here is a clear reason why one should be giving pyrazinamide intermittently. The point is that pyrazinamide blocks the excretion of uric acid. If you give it three times a week, there is a sufficiently long period between the doses for the excess uric acid to be excreted, and if I were having modern chemotherapy, I would want my pyrazinamide to be given intermittently, even if the other drugs were being given daily. In fact, in the Hong Kong study in which pyrazinamide was being given daily, three times a week, or twice a week, the incidence of arthralgia was 1 per cent when

---

[130] Dr David Girling wrote: 'This programme of research is reported in: O'Mahoney and Wing-kar (1973). See also Worlledge (1973a, 1973b).' Letter to Dr Daphne Christie, 8 April 2005.

[131] Mudie *et al.* (1954).

it was being given twice a week, 3 per cent when it was being given three times a week, and 7 per cent when it was being given daily. So the laboratory results correlated very nicely with the clinical studies.

Jindani: Just to give you the scale of the problem: in Study A we randomized 1355 patients to three short-course regimens, and in only 27 did we have to stop or change treatment because of adverse effects. Most of these were jaundice, but there were four cases of ocular side-effects due to ethambutol and the ethambutol had to be stopped. There was one case of thrombocytopaenic purpura and one patient had an isoniazid psychosis, but that was all.

Ormerod: People were concerned about giving three hepatotoxic drugs together, but in some of the US PHS (Public Health Service) studies of isoniazid prophylaxis, there was actually a placebo arm, and hepatitis occurred in 0.7 per cent of the placebo group, so in certain parts of the world with poorer sanitation we have to remember some of the so-called drug hepatitis may just be hepatitis A, hepatitis B, or hepatitis C, and that the placebo had a hepatitis rate.

Girling: I think one of the best studies of isoniazid versus placebo as chemoprophylaxis was the one from Finland, wasn't it, with Riska? He had well over 30 000 subjects randomized to isoniazid or placebo, and showed that the added risk of hepatitis from isoniazid was only 5.2 per 1000 subjects per year.[132] So that was isoniazid on its own. Then, of course, there was a great worry, as you say, when you add rifampicin and pyrazinamide. I think there are quite good reasons for thinking that rifampicin might not be hepatotoxic. Certainly, in our trial in Hong Kong, in which silicotic patients were given prophylaxis with isoniazid or rifampicin or isoniazid plus rifampicin or placebo, there was virtually no hepatotoxicity with rifampicin alone. There was a little with isoniazid, and with isoniazid and rifampicin.

Angel: I think one of the reasons that it got its reputation was because originally it was used very much as a second- or even third-line drug, and it was used on patients who were in pretty bad condition, a lot of them heavy drinkers. So there was quite a lot of underlying liver disease, I think, in the patients who were given rifampicin.

Girling: Of course, it was given in high dosages too.

Crofton: One of the peculiar things about this is that you can then go back and give the drug again afterwards, and that seems rather surprising. I don't

---

[132] Riska (1976).

know whether any expert toxicologists can explain this. Is it just that the liver is not very sensitive? It doesn't occur if you give the drug again.

Girling: Can anyone help us on that? It's certainly been our experience in trials that you can use the same regimen again, and, of course, what did, I think, confuse some people was that it's quite usual to get an increase in serum transaminase concentrations during the early weeks of antituberculosis chemotherapy anyway, and that these just come down again.

Angel: Sometimes you will see transaminase zoom up before you start treatment.

Davies: The Americans have invented their own weapon of mass destruction called pyrazinamide and rifampicin alone for people who are fit and well, but just happen to have a positive skin test. I have just been asked to review a paper that shows that RZ (rifampin and pyrazinamide) has a greater hepatotoxicity than HRZ (isoniazid, rifampin and pyrazinamide).[133]

Mitchison: Can I explain how that regimen got into being, because it's actually quite interesting? It was because of some mouse experiments done by Jacques Grosset, who is normally one of the most careful, thorough people, but he never looked at blood levels of drugs in his mice, and we showed a little bit later that unlike in man, you get interference in absorption of drugs, and that some of the effects that he thought were drug–drug interaction, were in fact due to differences in drug absorption.[134] He found the regimen that was best was this RZ regimen, but it was because of a drug absorption problem, and didn't therefore really apply in man. Rick O'Brien, who was in charge then of starting preventive chemotherapy studies,[135] took up this wonderful new regimen with great enthusiasm and despite adverse comments [verbal] from Wallace Fox and myself.[136] I remember very clearly the meeting at which it happened – this RZ regimen was promulgated in the USA, and it has done a great deal of damage in my view. But this is just a very sad example of failure at the more fundamental level in the mouse work leading to a bad mistake at the clinical level.

---

[133] See Girling (1978).

[134] Dickinson *et al.* (1992).

[135] See American Thoracic Society/Centers for Disease Control and Prevention/Infectious Diseases Society of America (2003).

[136] See Mitchison (1990); O'Brien (1989).

Ormerod: The hepatitis rate with that combination is 6.5 per cent, because I have had to review it for something I am doing for the Joint Tuberculosis Committee at the moment, with a high fatality rate as well. On this side of the Atlantic, we were getting our guidelines together at much the same time. We said we would not use it because it was going to be more toxic, it was no more effective than 3RH and there wasn't a combination tablet available for RZ, whereas there is for RH, so you still wouldn't guarantee people weren't taking monotherapy. I am afraid we were proved right on this side of the pond. But we are not having an inquiry about it.

Girling: Any more points about drug toxicity? Those of you in clinical practice have on the whole, I assume, found the modern short-course chemotherapy to be very acceptable to patients and not unduly toxic, which is what we certainly found in our trials.

Campbell: David, there's one theoretical thing that strikes me that's different over the last ten to 15 years, compared with 20 to 30 years ago. Many patients are on many different drugs by the time they get to 55, and we did the same trials, you did and the BTA did, in populations that were not very likely to be taking other drugs. Now in this country, I don't know about Scandinavia and Europe and the USA, practically everybody is on treatment for hypertension; they are taking their thiazide, they may be taking an ACE [angiotensin-converting enzyme] inhibitor. I think it's well worth ongoing surveillance, looking at side-effects, because of the poly-pharmacy that exists today.

Ormerod: Just to reply to that. That is getting less and less of a problem in the UK, nearly 70 per cent of patients are now non-white, and the median age of those patients is 29. The white population's median age is 55 so it is only a minority of the white population with tuberculosis who tend to be below 50. So that's 15 per cent of the cohort are likely to be on aspirin, statins, ACE inhibitors, the super pill that was talked about. The majority of people with tuberculosis are not on things for the other chronic diseases in the UK at the moment.

Meadway: But it's very different in Africa, where a large proportion of patients with tuberculosis will have HIV. In KwaZulu–Natal the incidence of HIV positivity is 26 per cent, I think, in adults. It will be higher in tuberculosis patients – 80 per cent.[137] So you are really dealing with a population who, if they are being treated appropriately, will by definition be on something else and will

---

[137] See, for example, Wilkinson and Moore (1996).

need the something else to recover fully from their tuberculosis and to prevent relapse. So when we are looking at the evidence that people have gathered through the years about the different toxicities of the different drugs, that's something that we are going to need to draw on when looking to the future for planning the appropriate treatment for those patients. It's very interesting, it seems to be rifampicin which showed up as less hepatotoxic than some of the others, because often rifampicin is the very one that interacts and cannot be used with antiretrovirals. That's the opposite of what one would have wanted. Looking back at the research that's been done, not in HIV patients, and not in patients with poly-pharmacy, that's going to be the pointer for the future, isn't it, to work out where to go next with these very difficult situations.

Dr Elizabeth Hills: With regard to toxicity. There was a problem with isoniazid in Tanzania, because they use the tablets that are 150 mg of rifampicin with 100 mg of isoniazid, and so if people need 600 mg of rifampicin they are getting 400 mg of isoniazid, and there were quite a lot of problems with peripheral neuropathy. Admittedly, some of them may have got HIV as well, that may contribute to it, I don't know. But also a problem in that you couldn't necessarily get the pyridoxine to treat them, so that was a problem. As I listen to this, and thinking about it, I think that there are more side-effects in a place like Tanzania, than possibly have been reported in the trials, because in many cases the drugs are being administered by people with rather minimal medical training. Sometimes they were rural medical aides in the past, they are gradually being upgraded over the years, but people who are just not aware of what the side-effects are. If you have got a fever you have got malaria, or if you have got a bit of jaundice, you have probably got malaria. People would be allowed to get extremely ataxic with their streptomycin without anybody doing anything about it. So I think we don't really know the incidence of side-effects in East Africa perhaps.

Darbyshire: It's actually true, we used to do some comparisons, David [Girling] and I, of the side-effects between the African trials, and the Hong Kong and Singapore trials. There were definitely much lower reported rates of toxicity in the African trials.[138]

---

[138] Girling (1989); For trials relating to thiacetazone see East African/[British] Medical Research Council (1960, 1963); Hong Kong Antituberculosis Association and Government Tuberculosis Association/[British] Medical Research Council (1968). For a more general article see Miller *et al.* (1972).

Mitchison: Perhaps I should say something here about the isoniazid toxicity studies that were done in Madras, because they are actually a beautiful example of a highly investigated problem, with very clearcut answers. What happened was that there was a big study in Madras with isoniazid alone, at different dose sizes, largely because WHO wanted to know what would happen with treatment with isoniazid.[139] Then following that, there were some further studies of high-dosage isoniazid in which glutamic acid, B group vitamins and so on, were added. These showed quite conclusively that it was vitamin B6 that was necessary both to stop and to some extent to cure peripheral neuropathy. And they also showed that there was a marked dosage effect.[140] Now from these studies we showed that the incidence of peripheral neuropathy is determined by the area under the curve (total exposure) of isoniazid, whereas the efficacy of isoniazid is determined by the peak isoniazid concentration, due to the selection of resistant mutants.[141] That was a beautiful set of results, I think probably one of the best pharmacological and clinical investigations ever done. At the end, 2 mg of vitamin B6 prevented peripheral neuropathy, so it shouldn't be very expensive.

Crofton: How much was the incidence related to malnutrition? I mean, poor slum dwellers in Madras and a lot of Africans are very malnourished. Did you get a higher amount of neuropathy in the malnourished than the others, or did you make any studies of that?

Mitchison: Wallace did a study on the food intake of the patients, but I don't think it established a relationship with neuropathy. I think all that it really did was to establish that the Madras population had a vitamin B-deficient diet, and therefore at the 300 mg isoniazid dose level, you probably were wise to give a small B6 supplement.[142] If you were using higher dosages, it was really very necessary. So there was a look at dietary factors, it was quite a thorough investigation done with the ICMR (Indian Council of Medical Research) nutritional unit.[143] Anyway it didn't actually correlate peripheral neuropathy with diet.

---

[139] Tuberculosis Chemotherapy Centre, Madras (1960).

[140] Tuberculosis Chemotherapy Centre, Madras (1963a, 1963b).

[141] Mitchison (1973): 171–82.

[142] Ramakrishnan *et al.* (1966).

[143] For a review, see, for example, Jawahar (2004).

Crofton: It's rather a subsidiary aspect of this, but I know that in the current National Tuberculosis Programmes of India and Malawi, they have been rather concerned with the number of deaths in sputum-negative patients with tuberculosis, and there's been a lot of discussion as to whether this may be due to malnutrition, because they are often very malnourished. But it's extremely difficult to work out an ethical controlled trial, keeping some people malnourished and doing things to others, and you might do it by giving specific vitamins, but perhaps people who are engaged in these researches now might comment on that.

Ormerod: I am not involved in research there, but a very high proportion of these people are likely to be HIV-positive and I think that's the explanation.

Hills: And also as they are sputum-negative, and in these countries you have not got any very accurate diagnostic methods, they have often got some other pulmonary disease. In many countries I think they are beginning to realize now, but they had been saying they didn't see pneumocystis. There are other conditions and it may not have been tuberculosis.

Girling: Shall we move on to preventing drug resistance, and I think Peter Davies is going to introduce this topic for us.

Davies: Thank you, David. I think in the UK we have actually been very good, by and large, at preventing the emergence of drug resistance. Certainly, as I was a senior house officer, registrar and a consultant through to about 1990, it really didn't impinge on my practice. There are papers published by the MRC, which show drug resistance varying between 4 and 7 per cent for isoniazid alone, but certainly MDR (multidrug-resistant) tuberculosis wasn't very much of a problem until about 1993.[144] I will come to that in a second, but I think there are three ways in the UK in which we have been able to ensure that drug resistance has been a minor or a lesser problem.

First of all, by ensuring compliance. We have done this, again, in three ways. Tuberculosis health visitors have been mentioned already. Ken [Citron] brought them up in the 1960s and these have formed a vital link between the hospital, the clinician and the patient, and I think if we didn't have tuberculosis health visitors we would have a big drug resistance problem. Countries that do not have had drug resistance problems, and areas of this country that have not had them, have had drug resistance problems. In Liverpool by fighting and

[144] See, for example, Adegbola *et al.* (2003).

fighting and fighting, we've got our allocation of tuberculosis health visitors, one to 40 and we have got our clerical support, but dotted all around, satellites to Liverpool, are places which do not have tuberculosis health visitors and they are a right pain, they really are. Unless we get our health visitors, tuberculosis visitors, right the way round, doing their work in adequate numbers, we are going to have this potential for drug resistance. But I think tuberculosis health visitors have formed the mainstay in preventing drug resistance over the last 40 years in the UK.

Secondly, selective DOTS has been very important. Those patients that really do not comply at home taking their own medication have had to go on DOTS. We have been using that selectively in the UK, I would say with pretty good effect.

Thirdly, physician control. It is important that there is a chest physician who is in command of an area and has overall control to make sure that health visitors do their stuff, and that the patients are therefore seen to be doing their stuff. So that's three subheadings under the heading ensuring compliance: tuberculosis visitors, selective DOTS and physician control.

The second important ingredient for preventing the emergence of drug resistance, I believe, is fixed-dose combination (FDC) chemotherapy, which we have used traditionally in this country ever since I started, that's 30 years. I did a study once comparing the use of FDCs in the UK with the USA. This is going back ten years. In 1993 75 per cent of all rifampicin prescribed in this country was attached to isoniazid, or isoniazid and pyrazinamide, 75 per cent of all rifampicin was in FDCs, and this must have included rifampicin given in preventive therapy as well. So that's good. My colleague in the USA couldn't find accurate figures, but it was certainly no better than 20 per cent and was probably about 11 per cent. They have had big problems with emergent MDR in the USA. If you look at the figures on the website for HPA (Health Protection Agency) you will find that MDR began to emerge as a problem in the UK in about 1993. It was 0.6 per cent then and that was the first year that I had my MDR patients. It then climbed to 1.7 per cent in 1996, it has gone down a little, and it's gone up a little. My feeling is that what we are getting now is basically imported. What we had in 1993 was largely self-inflicted.

There's one further area that I would like to bring up as a controversial point here, and that is the introduction of HRZ as opposed to HRE or HRZE as a possible potential for creating drug resistance, in that Z is less good at preventing the emergence of drug resistance compared with E. So bringing in Z as the third drug on its own might possibly have been a contributing factor.

There's an editorial on this in *Chest*; around about that date, querying it.[145] There's absolutely no proof, it's very hypothetical, but it does seem to be a relatively interesting coincidence in terms of time and the development of the relatively few MDR cases we have had. So that's what I want to say about preventing the emergence of drug resistance, finishing up on a controversial note.

Meadway: I agree totally with what you say, but I would love to pick up on two things. One was that the thing that helped prevent drug resistance emerging was a combination tablet of two effective antituberculosis drugs, and the other was that in the UK we do have a certain amount of resistance already and much of our tuberculosis is imported. Take those two together and you have a significant proportion of people with tuberculosis who have isoniazid resistance before you start. You tend to find that out at the end of a couple of months of treatment, by which time the patient has been taking a combination of rifampicin and isoniazid, which acts as one drug because isoniazid their tuberculosis is resistant to, and two other drugs that are also separate tablets quite often, and they sometimes pick and choose. I had a patient who picked and chose.[146] She had HIV but she had tuberculosis. Her initial culture was isoniazid resistant, which we didn't know, of course, at the onset. She picked and chose which of her drugs she took and took them rather intermittently, and by the time she had treatment failure and pyrexia, and wasn't responding, her cultures showed multidrug-resistant, rifampicin-resistant tuberculosis. So my question is why are we being so slow about asking and pressing for a combination tablet of something other than rifampicin and isoniazid, because isn't that what we need in isoniazid resistance?

Davies: The answer is, yes we do. We have Rifater, rifampicin/isoniazid/ pyrazinamide and we have a potential of licensing of a four-drug combination called 'Rimcure', but unfortunately, that has yet to be licensed. That's the four drugs in one tablet, and they have certainly got that in many other countries. I cannot help the name, I didn't invent that.

Ormerod: Are you talking about the continuation phase? What we need is Bac Tec rapid culture methods everywhere, or access to them, so that by the time

---

[145] Kahana (1996). See also Kritski *et al.* (1997).

[146] Dr Jeannette Meadway wrote: 'An African woman living in East London'. E-mail to Dr Daphne Christie 21 April 2005.

that you get to two months, you have got the organism and you have got the sensitivity data. Then you can have a proper continuation phase, and if somebody has got drug resistance it can be monitored. The problem is with only 6 per cent isoniazid monoresistance in the UK you are not going to get somebody who will make you a combination of rifampicin/ethambutol, but the key to preventing it is giving a four-drug initial combination, because of the populations that we have. We are not alone. The American Thoracic Society (ATS) says with 4 per cent isoniazid resistance you should use a four-drug combination, the European Respiratory Society (ERS) says 2 per cent. But the answer is getting your bacteriological confirmation, which needs people to send the samples, plus faster culture and faster susceptibility data.

Meadway: I agree 100 per cent with everything you said. The point about it is that Rifater, when you look at what the patients have got to swallow, having those big tablets is difficult, and the number that they have to take, and to try to persuade an HIV patient on loads of other medication to take Rifater is much more difficult than to persuade them to take Rifinah equivalent plus the pyrazinamide separately. Plus they can jiggle around the times of rifampicin and pyrazinamide to be different and therefore easier to take if they are in separate medications. So the very patient, who isn't likely to cooperate by adhering to their medication, is the very one who is going to object to taking a handful of Rifater. So I don't think the triple and quadruple combinations in the induction phase will solve the problem with that type of patient who had poor adherence to medication because they find them difficult to take.

Moore-Gillon: If I can step back to the period being covered by the seminar, and it's something which Peter [Davies] talked about, which was physician compliance with these recommended regimens, and I wonder if I can ask the people who were around at the time about the role of the BTA and the Thoracic Society, and crucially about the enmity which I am told existed between the BTA and the Thoracic Society. Did this really happen, or is this a figment of my boss's imagination when I was a junior doctor?

Citron: Can I reserve that for my contribution?

Crofton: Just one slight historical point. Knut Øvreberg and I were at, I think, the second meeting of WHO when they took on tuberculosis in a big way in the early 1990s and there was a long discussion as to what should be done widely. In that discussion, the whole day, there wasn't a word about resistance, so we wrote a joint memorandum and said they really must pay attention to this, they must get some idea of how severe a problem this was internationally.[147] Of course, they have done very good surveys since.

Can I make one other clinical point? There's a general feeling in the world that the word of God comes out of laboratories, and it's only clinicians who make mistakes. In many countries I have been asked to see a patient, 'We have just had results showing drug resistance, and what are we going to do?'. You go through the story of this patient; he's responded perfectly well to chemotherapy, they've just got a report from the lab. They never think of asking the bacteriologist down to discuss it. So do remember that mistakes occur in laboratories too.

Citron: Referring back to this isoniazid-resistant HIV-positive patient. I think there's evidence that HIV-positive patients, at least in this country, have more pretreatment isoniazid resistance than HIV-negative patients. Remember that you can request a gene probe for rifampicin resistance, and you will get the answer back in 48 hours. Now something like over 90 per cent of pretreatment rifampicin-resistant organisms are also isoniazid resistant too, so I think that you can select patients for this gene probe, which can be done in the central laboratory and you will get your answer within 48 hours.

Chalmers: I want to ask a question and then place something on the record. I think John Crofton will probably be able to answer the question best. The MRC trial of streptomycin for pulmonary tuberculosis is justifiably celebrated as a methodological landmark in research.[148] One of the things that people say, is that it was important because it revealed the development of resistance, and indeed documented the eighth nerve damage that you can get with streptomycin. So my question is, to what extent is that trial seen in that light as a particularly important contribution?

---

[147] See Crofton and Øvreberg (1992). Unpublished Memorandum in WHO. Sir John Crofton wrote: '*Summary*: Much anecdotal, but little systematic, evidence that drug resistance may be an important barrier to an effective National Tuberculosis Programme in certain countries, notably in Asia. *Technical problems*: Methods should be reviewed and standardization attained to ensure tests in different laboratories are comparable. *Determining extent of problem*: Sample surveys in relevant countries of "newly presenting" and "retreatment" patients. *Potential causes of resistance and potential remedies*: Outlined. *Expert Committee*: Proposed. All these suggestions were later very well taken up by WHO.' Letter to Dr Daphne Christie, 28 March 2005.

[148] Chalmers (2005). Sir John Crofton wrote: 'It is worth remembering that streptomycin was the first new important antibiotic after penicillin. Patients on penicillin did not develop resistance under treatment. Patients on streptomycin did. This was a grim new phenomenon.' Letter to Dr Daphne Christie, 28 March 2005.

The other thing that I wanted to mention, and to place on the record, relates to the reputation of the tuberculosis specialists in respect of the very systematic way that they have used randomized controlled trials to assess treatments. When Archie Cochrane judged which speciality in medicine deserved the gold medal for being the most evidence-based, he gave a 'Bradford' (a 'gold medal' named for Bradford Hill) to the tuberculosis specialists, and he gave my background speciality, obstetrics, the wooden spoon![149]

This view is not universal in respect to the tuberculosis specialists, however. About four years ago I met Christopher Murray, a very senior member of Bruntland's[150] [Gro Harlem Bruntland, Director-General] cabinet at WHO. I was trying to persuade him that WHO ought to take a more systematic approach to controlled randomized studies. On the basis of his belief that the Madras sanatorium study had actually resulted in the antibiotic resistance that people were now facing, he appeared to believe that all randomized controlled trials were deeply misleading. So it's an interesting contrast between the way that Archie Cochrane regarded your speciality, and the way that a senior member of WHO staff seems prepared to jettison everything about what you have done that I regard as important.

Mitchison: Can I make two methodological points about this whole programme? One of them is that no patient was excluded for initial drug resistance. This has been of tremendous value, because it is the only way that one can really assess the contribution made by a drug and, of course, how important it is to be able to measure drug resistance. I mean, here we have been talking about rapid diagnosis, and yet for most treatments isoniazid resistance has no effect at all on the prognosis of modern chemotherapy, whereas resistance to rifampicin does. One wouldn't know that sort of thing if one hadn't had that methodological decision. This was not available from any of the American studies; they always exclude everybody with resistance and so they are almost valueless for looking at the effects of individual drugs.

The second thing, just a minor comment really, and that was that there are much quicker and cheaper methods available now for getting very rapid sensitivity tests. Particularly the phage methods, which have been developed in various ways, are much quicker and much cheaper. The real problem you will

---

149 Cochrane (1979): 1–11.

150 Dr Christopher Murray was appointed Executive Director, Evidence and Information for Policy Cluster of the World Health Organization in May 2001.

have with a quick sensitivity test is that they tend to be based on expensive packaging in which some people are making a packet.

Girling: I think that's a very important point. I was looking back at the old results in Hong Kong; this was on the use of isoniazid and PAS for 18 months with streptomycin for the first two. There's quite a high level of drug resistance in Hong Kong, and even in patients with initial resistance to all three drugs, the treatment was successful in about 40 per cent, and that's even with the old regimen. Results in patients with initial isoniazid resistance were almost as good as in patients who were subsequently found to have fully susceptible strains. So resistance is a relative thing.

Mitchison: Very recent work, actually looking at the distribution of drug resistance inside the lungs, shows that what you actually see in the sputum can be completely different from the foci, bacillary foci, in the lungs, which often show very diverse patterns.[151] So the fact that we actually see resistant tubercle bacilli in the sputum does not necessarily imply that the same resistance patterns are present all through the lungs. It just means that sputum bacteriology is only a relative help, not an absolute help.

Crofton: I think it probably depends at what stage the resistance is developing. We found the same thing in the early days. But Iain Chalmers was asking about the first streptomycin trial. It's quite interesting, I recently looked back again at that report and Denny and I worked together at the Brompton, because I was coordinating the Brompton part of the trial, and of course it was streptomycin alone, and the original intention of the MRC was to treat the patients for six months, but because so much drug resistance occurred[152] and many of these patients relapsed when resistance did occur, the conclusion at the end of that was that chemotherapy could only be an accessory treatment, but then, of course, fortunately, the other drugs came on. It's quite interesting that the initial response to this famous trial was rather negative, until we got the other drugs.

Davies: To go back to what Iain [Chalmers] was saying about Chris Murray, I think he deserves three or four marks out of ten. The lesson of Madras was that patients under close supervision, being treated at home, did just as well as those in sanatoria.[153] The word there is close supervision. Now what's

---

[151] Kaplan *et al.* (2003).

[152] Crofton and Mitchison (1948).

[153] Tuberculosis Chemotherapy Centre, Madras (1959).

happened as a result is people say patients do just as well at home as they do in sanatoria so send them home with the drugs and they will do fine. And of course that is not learning the lesson of Madras. The lesson of Madras is close supervision. So in a sense, Madras has given people the wrong, well they have taken the wrong message out of Madras, and that could well be contributing to drug resistance. So I think Chris Murray deserves three out of ten. But he's a young lad, he's done a lot and he deserves to be re-educated, and I would welcome him back.

Angel: Apropos of Denny's last remarks, in the chronic trial, the chronic MRC trial,[154] where we took patients with quite big cavities and treated them for one year, two years, or three years, we did get a group with what was labelled isolated positive cultures, and quite often these were resistant, but then you carried on the treatment and you had no further trouble. So this may have been the sort of sample of stuff from the cavity wall.

Girling: Our last topic is implementing short-course therapy in routine clinical practice, and I think Ken is going to start us off on this, and then I think Amina [Jindani] might perhaps chip in with something on developing countries, if we are still allowed to call them that.

Citron: Thank you, David. What I want to do is to try to give an overall impression of the way that short-course chemotherapy was introduced into routine clinical practice in England and Wales. I want to start in the 1960s, and early 1970s when, as I said, we were using isoniazid and PAS for 18 months to two years, with streptomycin initially. This was routine practice, in hospitals and in chest clinics, and I have already mentioned that we published our follow-up in 1971 and we were delighted because 90 per cent of patients were treated for the allocated time and all but 2 per cent became culture-negative, and on a follow-up for three to seven years none of those actually relapsed. So we were happy. Now there were a lot of other physicians who were also very happy, because physicians on the whole tend to be rather conservative, with a little 'c', and they tend to persist in using regimens with which they are familiar. Of course, not all these physicians ever counted their failures, and this was a problem that they got the impression that they were doing very well, but they hadn't actually had a prolonged follow-up.

The other point I think was that they weren't going to change to new-fangled regimens which they had read about and had been studied in Africa and in

---

[154] Medical Research Council/Tuberculosis Chemotherapy Trials Committee (1962).

Hong Kong and so on, they wanted to have something for British patients, English and Welsh patients living here, which they regarded probably as very different. I am talking about England and Wales. I am not talking about Scotland, which was managed by John Crofton. Remember, and we must keep on stressing this, that we had a very adequate number of tuberculosis nurses, so that we had the ability for close supervision at that time. I think that there was a general feeling, especially among the old chest physicians, who had seen tuberculosis patients lying about in sanatoria for years, to regard tuberculosis as something that needed very prolonged treatment. They had seen a number of apparently wonderful breakthroughs like gold therapy[155] and they had seen all that fail, so there was a great deal of scepticism, at that time. I have no doubt that the studies that were done by the BTTA, as it was then called, were a very important factor in convincing physicians to adopt these short-course regimens.[156] Now, as Joe [Angel] has said, the first BTA study was started in 1972. It was run by a committee and the coordinators were Joe Angel and Alan Somner, and at various times, Ian Campbell and Tony Dyson. I was chairing the committee. The statistics were done by Ian Sutherland,[157] and I am very sorry that Ian isn't well enough to be here this afternoon. The mycobacteriology was done by Joe Selkon.[158] I won't go over the details, but will just remind you this was a big study. We had over 900 patients admitted to the study.[159] They were divided into eight regimens, and these were rifampicin and isoniazid for six months, nine months, 12 months, or 18 months, and allocated to either streptomycin or ethambutol for two months initially.

In 1976 we published the results with a two-year post-treatment follow-up, which showed 100 per cent conversion and no relapse in the nine-month regimen.[160] Because ethambutol was easier to take than streptomycin, the BTTA recommended that EHR [ethambutol, isoniazid, rifampicin] for nine months was the optimal treatment.

---

[155] See Benedek (2004).

[156] See note 91.

[157] Dr Ian Sutherland was Director of the Medical Research Council's Statistical Research and Services Unit in 1969. See Sutherland (1998): 2554–62.

[158] See Tony Jenkins comment on page 70.

[159] Dr Joseph Angel wrote: '911, actually.' Note on draft transcript, 27 July 2004.

[160] British Thoracic and Tuberculosis Association (1976).

At that time I had the great pleasure of associating with Wallace Fox. He was the most practical clinician you could meet and he was very concerned with what was actually happening in practice in England and Wales, and he talked about, as I think has been mentioned, physician compliance, or lack of physician compliance with recommended regimens. With his MRC study team, he looked at the epidemiology of tuberculosis throughout the UK. That study was done in 1978–9, two or three years after the official BTTA pronouncement of optimal therapy. He studied the treatment that was actually given rather than what physicians said they gave. In fact, what was found was that only one-third of patients were having anything like the BTTA recommended regimen and most patients, at least half, were having very long periods of treatment. So physicians were really very reluctant to reduce treatment duration to nine months.[161]

You have already heard about the strong prejudice against pyrazinamide there was at that time, because many physicians had seen toxicity in drug-resistant cases given high doses of pyrazinamide for a prolonged period of time. It was regarded as a dangerous drug. The BTTA did a national study of pyrazinamide given for the first two months with either ethambutol or streptomycin. The regimens were rifampicin and isoniazid for six months with pyrazinamide for the first two months, with either streptomycin or ethambutol. I have to say, and Joe Angel will remember this, that there were a few very eminent physicians who said they wouldn't cooperate because we were using this dangerous drug, pyrazinamide. It was a very closely supervised study, we were doing routine liver function tests frequently throughout. We found that there was no difference in the incidence of hepatitis or the results of liver function tests between the pyrazinamide regimens and the non-pyrazinamide-containing control regimen, so that we were able to reassure physicians that it was safe given in this dose for this period of time. In 1982 we published a two-year post-treatment follow-up, which showed that the six-month regimen was as good as the nine-month.[162] The regimen of six months' rifampicin and isoniazid with initial pyrazinamide and ethambutol was recommended by the British Thoracic Society for use in Britain in 1984.[163] The MRC published the Singapore results in 1981, and the East and Central African study was in 1983, so we published, as it were, in the middle of these two very important MRC papers.

---

[161] Medical Research Council Tuberculosis and Chest Diseases Unit (1985).

[162] British Thoracic Association (1982).

[163] British Thoracic Society (1984).

I am quite sure that these multicentre studies were the thing that gave our physicians' confidence in and experience of using short-course chemotherapy, and I think that these BTTA studies transformed clinical research into practical benefits for patients. Unfortunately, I cannot tell you how quickly the six-month recommendation was taken up, because, very sadly, the MRC Tuberculosis and Chest Diseases Unit was shut down in 1986 when Wallace retired and it wasn't possible to do that study. But I am sure we have data now to show how this has become the standard treatment.[164]

Dr Tony Jenkins: I would have to correct Ken [Citron] slightly.[165] Joe Selkon provided bacteriological advice to the committee, but it was my laboratory that did all the bacteriology for both studies, and that brings me to another point. The volume of work, particularly at the intake period, was enormous. Specimens were flooding into the laboratory in great numbers. As one of the staff so eloquently put it, 'We are drowning in a sea of spit'. Fortunately we had the capacity to absorb that amount of work, but the staff were working their socks off to do it. The second study also involved routine urine testing for isoniazid metabolites. My point is that to get that sort of study done today, from the laboratory point of view, I don't think you could do it in the UK, I don't think there is a laboratory that could handle that volume of primary work, and I don't think the accountants would let us do it. Somebody would have to pay, and that work didn't cost the BTTA, it cost the PHLS [Public Health Laboratory Service] in one way, but it was absorbed totally through the PHLS budget, but today it would be quite a different ball game.

Girling: Amina, do you want to add anything on implementing short-course chemotherapy in developing countries, particularly in African countries?

Jindani: Yes, I want to repeat that our experiences – and I think Andrew, Janet, Denny will confirm this – in Africa and other countries where we did trials, things were quite different to your experiences in that our colleagues wholeheartedly embraced short-course chemotherapy. Imagine 18 months to six months, wow! They wholeheartedly embraced it. They have a great deal of confidence and will accept almost anything. This can be a disadvantage, because in a country like Nepal for instance, there are about 3000 NGOs, local and overseas, operating in Nepal, not all in tuberculosis, but this is the extent

---

[164] Ormerod and Prescott (2003).

[165] See page 68.

of interference if you like. So we have the Japanese in the east saying use this regimen, the Germans in the middle saying use this, and the Brits in the west. Everybody's getting a mixed message and so there is no standard chemotherapy – and this is not just Nepal, this is in many other countries – so on the one hand, while this is an advantage to have such cooperating, collaborating compliant colleagues, on the other hand it can be a disadvantage.

Booth: First, I have to confess I was chairman of the MRC Tropical Medicine Research Board that, in fact, made the decision that Wallace Fox should not be replaced when he retired. That's simply a confession. Second point, having listened with such interest to Ken Citron's presentation, what does that mean in terms of health service provision now in 2004? Who treats tuberculosis, is it chest physicians, is it infectious diseases doctors? Do cardiologists treat tuberculous pericarditis, do gastroenterologists treat tuberculosis of the gut? What is the answer to that? My third question is that after 50 years having been through so many different studies – and we have heard a lot about very many of them today – does the National Institute for Clinical Excellence now give advice to the health service on precisely what they should do with patients with tuberculosis?

Ormerod: I will answer. I will follow on Ken's comments about who treats what and how quickly it came in, and I will answer a number of those questions following it. When the MRC Tuberculosis Unit stopped being a tuberculosis unit, it became briefly the Cardiothoracic Epidemiology Group, which together with the BTS looked at the outcome of the 1988 survey, and subsequently we have looked at it. So 11 per cent of people got short-course chemotherapy of six months in 1983, and it was up to over 80 per cent by 1988, and now it's very exceptional if people don't get that. But what people give is often longer than seven months, because we allow five to seven months as a wide range, and people are still being treated for too long, not everybody gets fixed-dose combinations, and in the last survey in 1998, we could only demonstrate that about 60 per cent had actually got proper compliance monitoring. So that's to say what's happening. Chest physicians treat 85 per cent of tuberculosis in this country for pulmonary and nonpulmonary; infectious disease physicians treat 4 per cent; cardiologists I hope treat nothing, because they know nothing about tuberculosis, and chest physicians statistically are better at sticking to recommendations than all other groups, including infectious disease physicians. B category data were published in the *Royal College of Physicians Journal* following the 1993 survey, we also showed it after the 1998 survey, but we couldn't include it in the paper because I think it had been refereed by an infectious disease physician.[166]

Girling: So it was a matter of the BTS rather than NICE?

Ormerod: No, the BTS last produced guidelines on chemotherapy and management in 1998, and on contact tracing, control and prevention in 2000.[167] These are currently being looked at by NICE; the Royal College of Physicians' Clinical Effectiveness Unit is handling this and I am the clinical adviser, along with other members in this room, to that process, which started on 17 December and will go through for about 18 months before gestation occurs.

Darbyshire: I just wanted to follow on from Tony Jenkins' comment about sputum, because the thing I remember about the studies in East Africa and Hong Kong is jumbo jets full of sputum flying in from Hong Kong and I think that it's important that we acknowledge Bryan Allen, who actually masterminded that whole venture, and Terry Morris, who made sure that they arrived off the airplane and got to the Hammersmith in time. Because it was again another difference between Hong Kong in that we had technicians, I think, seconded from your unit, Denny, into Kenya, Tanzania and Zambia, with Eric, John and Aidan. When I took over, when the Unit did close, and I remember that day very well, I was taken to Heathrow through all the back roads and shown where the specimens arrived, because if there was a crisis, I was going to be called to sort it out.

Angel: I would like to come to the defence of British clinicians, because when we proposed the first study, there was enormous enthusiasm among the clinicians who attended the BTTA summer meeting, and over the next seven months we had 911 patients and that was partly the reason for Tony Jenkins drowning in sputum. Similarly, with the second study, although there were some physicians who expressed grave doubts about the toxicity, hepatotoxicity, nevertheless we had 593 patients within a period of 18 months, so it was obviously slower than the first one, but still quite useful.

Crofton: Can I just say something about another form of conservatism internationally? In 1983 the IUATLD and WHO had a symposium in

---

[166] See Ormerod and Prescott (2003). Professor Ormerod wrote: 'The Scottish Intercollegiate Guidelines Network (SIGN) in 1998 were giving three gradings for evidence: A, metaanalysis or controlled trials; B, good clinical studies and C, nonevidence-based statements.' Note on draft transcript, 1 April 2005.

[167] Joint Tuberculosis Committee of the British Thoracic Society (2000).

Zimbabwe to try to have all the southern African countries there and to make recommendations about treatment. I was asked to chair the symposium and, with Karel Styblo, to write the report and recommendations. It was regarded as urgent. The symposium recommended that the countries should switch to short-course chemotherapy. Karel and I worked almost nonstop for 48 hours because of the alleged urgency, but then its publication and distribution were delayed for months and months by WHO because WHO thought that short-course drugs were too expensive for poor countries.[168] Later, when we introduced short-course chemotherapy through the Britain–Nepal Medical Trust with a trial comparing similar districts still using previous long-term treatment, we did a cost–benefit analysis. Rifampicin was still very expensive. But when we looked at the cost per cured patient, it was just the same as standard chemotherapy.[169]

Chalmers: In the 1970s and early 1980s how much tuberculosis research and tuberculosis programme delivery was funded by private donations, rich ex-patients or business corporations and charities?

Mitchison: Could I say something just on that one point about funding? You see, as far as the MRC funding was going, there was core funding for Wallace's unit, my unit, and this amounted at that time to about £1 million per annum, which of course would be quite a lot more now, but it still seemed quite small because it covered not just one study, but several studies going on simultaneously. There was also money coming in from what was then the Overseas Development Agency, which provided a special block of money allocated for this work. It was mainly used to promote the African studies. There was probably a bit of private donation money in the Hong Kong studies, because private money was used, for instance, to fund the laboratory building in Hong Kong. On the whole, the contribution in Britain was really very small from private funds.

Now the other point. I went over to the USA in about I suppose 1973 to present for the first time the results of short-course studies to the American Thoracic Society at their annual meeting. This was very interesting. I wasn't used to talking to large American meetings. It was at the end of a four-day conference, when you normally didn't have many people coming, but a big

[168] Sir John Crofton wrote: 'I think our report was only distributed by WHO in typescript.' Letter to Dr Daphne Christie, 28 March 2005.

[169] See Murray *et al.* (1990, 1991). See also Baker (1975).

ballroom entirely packed with very hostile people – that's what it was. I had to get up and put over these early clinical trials, and I was attacked right, left and centre. How could you do these unethical studies? How could you treat your patients for such a short time? One could answer back saying, 'Well, it's unethical to treat them for longer, you see.' But it was really quite unlike the situation in Africa unfortunately. You were met with terrible hostility because it came essentially from something outside their country. And, of course, coming from the old colonial master, which makes it even worse.

Girling: I think we have had an enormously enjoyable meeting, and I think we are now to be subjected to some fully supervised alcohol, with, we hope, not too many adverse effects.

Dr Daphne Christie: On behalf of the History of Twentieth Century Medicine Group, I would like to thank you for participating in today's seminar and to add our particular thanks to Dr David Girling for his excellent chairing of the meeting this afternoon.

Appendix 1

Wallace Fox's contributions to tuberculosis: Two memoirs[170]

Domiciliary chemotherapy and fully supervised intermittent regimens are the main pillars of today's global tuberculosis programme. Both these revolutionary concepts originated over four decades ago at the MRC Tuberculosis Chemotherapy Centre in Madras, during the stewardship of Wallace Fox. While this fact is fairly well known, the trying circumstances under which a randomized controlled trial of home and sanatorium treatment was undertaken are not documented. At the time, the prophets of doom were many, some saying that randomization was an alien concept in a developing country such as India, while others predicted that no patient could be confined to sanatorium for a year or expected to self-administer drugs at home daily for long periods. To persuade sanatorium patients to stay put, Fox visited them every week and discussed with his clinic staff the next morning any domestic problems arising from their hospitalization. To monitor compliance of patients treated at home, he introduced pill counts at periodic intervals and surprise urine tests to check on drug ingestion; also, home visits were made to retrieve defaulters, initially by health visitors/social workers and clinic doctors, and eventually by Fox himself! However, he was quick to realize that such heroic measures would be impracticable under routine programme conditions, and that alternative approaches were therefore necessary.

Fox's understanding of the problem of patient compliance was profound, as can be gleaned from his remarkable review in 1961 at the Amsterdam International Tuberculosis conference.[171] When he noticed that some patients on daily chemotherapy responded well despite minor degrees of irregularity, he wondered if less frequent chemotherapy but fully supervised, might not be equally effective, a concept suggested by studies of serial serum isoniazid concentrations in patients on daily chemotherapy. This was the rationale of the randomized control trial of fully supervised twice weekly treatment and self-administered daily treatment, and the successful outcome of this study, both

[170] These two tributes were written for this volume and sent from Mrs Wallace Fox to Dr Daphne Christie, 19 March 2005.

[171] Fox (1962b).

short-term and long-term, that was to become the genesis for the present day global DOTS strategy.

After five years at Madras, Fox returned to London in 1961. He could well have proclaimed then, like Julius Caesar did in 47 BC after vanquishing King Pontus in Asia Minor, 'Veni, Vidi, Vici' (I came, I saw, I conquered). There is no doubt that Fox put Madras on the tuberculosis map, but it is perhaps equally true that the Madras experience prepared him for stiffer challenges. Over the next three decades, even in the midst of his infinite commitments in East Africa, Hong Kong, Singapore, Czechoslovakia and the UK, he kept very close contact with the Madras Centre in all its research studies, notably of short-course regimens, through meticulous correspondence and annual consultant visits. Equally significant were his efforts in installing a serious research culture among national staff in Madras, and the building of a first rate infrastructure for tuberculosis research that will be celebrating its golden jubilee next year.

Thus, the facets of Fox's contributions to tuberculosis are many – pure science, infrastructure development and propagation of a good research culture in developing countries.

Dr S Radhakrishna, 2005

On his return in 1961 from secondment to India to establish and direct the Tuberculosis Chemotherapy Centre in Madras, Wallace rejoined the MRC Tuberculosis and Chest Diseases Unit at the Brompton Hospital, London, and was its director from 1965 until his retirement in 1986.

Under his inspired leadership, this unit conducted a hugely productive programme of randomized clinical trials and other epidemiological research in many countries, including the UK, Czechoslovakia, central and eastern Africa, Algeria, Hong Kong, Singapore, South Korea and Transkei. Moreover, collaborative research with the Tuberculosis Chemotherapy Centre, Madras, continued, and useful contributions were made to clinical trials methodology.

This programme of research identified highly effective treatment regimens for the successful management of smear-positive and smear-negative pulmonary tuberculosis, spinal tuberculosis, silicotuberculosis and tuberculous pericarditis. The problems of managing patients with initially drug-resistant disease and with acquired resistance were also addressed. Practical ways of supervising regimens, whether given daily or intermittently, were also developed. Wallace had a special interest in studying methods of supervising chemotherapy in a wide variety of local situations and so of maximizing patients' compliance in their treatment. Such patient populations included drug addicts and prisoners in Hong Kong, and Bedouin nomads in North Africa.

An important component of Wallace's research programme was studying adverse reactions to drug regimens and how best to prevent and treat them. His programme also led to the crucial demonstration of the high effectiveness of the combination of isoniazid, rifampicin and pyrazinamide, and so to the development of modern short-course (six-month) chemotherapy now universally accepted throughout the world. Few programmes of clinical research have had such an enormously beneficial impact on public health throughout the world; Wallace's contributions are universally acknowledged and appreciated.

Dr David Girling, 2004

References

Adegbola R A, Hill P, Baldeh I, Otu J, Sarr R, Sillah J, Lienhardt C, Corrah T, Manneh K, Drobniewski F, McAdam K P. (2003) Surveillance of drug-resistant *Mycobacterium tuberculosis* in The Gambia. *International Journal of Tuberculosis and Lung Disease* 7: 390–3.

Algerian Working Group/[British] Medical Research Council Cooperative Study. (1984) Controlled clinical trial comparing a 6-month and a 12-month regimen in the treatment of pulmonary tuberculosis in the Algerian Sahara. *American Review of Respiratory Disease* **129**: 921–8.

American Thoracic Society/Centers for Disease Control and Prevention/ Infectious Diseases Society of America. (2003) Treatment of tuberculosis. *American Journal of Respiratory and Critical Care Medicine* **167**: 603–62.

Angel J H, Citron K, Campbell I A, Somner A R. (1976) Short-course chemotherapy in pulmonary tuberculosis. *Bulletin of the International Union Against Tuberculosis* **51**: 57–60.

Anon. (1952) Notes and News: Isonicotinic acid derivatives in tuberculosis. *Lancet* **i**: 571.

Anon. (1977) Results at 5 years of a controlled comparison of a 6-month and a standard 18-month regimen of chemotherapy for pulmonary tuberculosis. *American Review of Respiratory Disease* **116**: 3–8.

Aquinas M. (1974) Observations on tuberculosis meningitis. *Bulletin of the International Union Against Tuberculosis* 49: 74–7.

Aronson J. (1999) When I use a word...That's show business. *British Medical Journal* **319**: 972.

Baker I A. (1975) The Britain–Nepal Medical Trust. *Annals of the Royal College of Surgeons of England* **57**: 48–9.

Barber M, Garrod L P. (eds) (1963) Streptomycin. Toxicity and side effects. *Antibiotic and Chemotherapy.* Chapter VI. Edinburgh: E & S Livingstone Ltd, 98–101.

Batten J. (1968) Experimental chemotherapy of tuberculosis. *British Medical Journal* **3**: 75–82.

Bayer R, Wilkinson D. (1995) Directly observed therapy for tuberculosis: History of an idea. *Lancet* **ii**: 1545–8.

Benedek T G. (2004) The history of gold therapy for tuberculosis. *Journal of the History of Medicine and Allied Sciences* **59**: 50–89.

Briggs I L, Rochester W R, Shennan D H. (1968) Streptomycin plus thiacetazone (Thioacetazone) compared with streptomycin plus PAS and with isoniazid plus thiacetazone in the treatment of pulmonary tuberculosis in Rhodesia. *Tubercle* **49**: 48–69.

Brindle R, Odhiambo J, Mitchison D. (2001) Serial counts of *Mycobacterium tuberculosis* in sputum as surrogate markers of the sterilising activity of rifampicin and pyrazinamide in treating pulmonary tuberculosis. *BMC Pulmonary Medicine* (electronic resource). **1**: 2. (www.biomedcentral.com/1471-2466/1/2) visited 28 June 2005.

British Thoracic Association. (1982) A controlled trial of 6 months chemotherapy in pulmonary tuberculosis. Second report: Results during the 24 months after the end of chemotherapy. *American Review of Respiratory Disease* **126**: 460–2.

British Thoracic Society. (1984) A controlled trial of 6 months' chemotherapy in pulmonary tuberculosis. Final report: Results during the 36 months after the end of chemotherapy and beyond. *British Journal of Diseases of the Chest* **78**: 330–6.

British Thoracic and Tuberculosis Association. (1975) Short-course chemotherapy in pulmonary tuberculosis. *Lancet* **i**: 119–24.

British Thoracic and Tuberculosis Association (1976) Short Course chemotherapy in pulmonary Tuberculosis. *Lancet* **ii**: 1102–4.

Brown I N, Glynn A A. (1987) The *Ity/Lsh/Bcg* gene significantly affects mouse resistance to *Mycobacterium lepraemurium. Immunology* **64**: 587–91.

Cairns H, Duthie E S, Smith H V. (1946) Intrathecal streptomycin in meningitis: Clinical trial in tuberculous, coliform and other infections. *Lancet* **ii**: 153–5.

Campbell I A, Dyson A J. (1977) Lymph node tuberculosis: A comparison of various methods of treatment. *Tubercle* **58**: 171–9.

Chalmers I. (2005) Statistical theory was not the reason that randomisation was used in the British Medical Research Council's clinical trial of streptomycin for pulmonary tuberculosis, in Weisz G, Jorland G, Opinerl A. (eds) *Quantification in the Medical and Health Sciences in Historical and Sociological Perspective.* Montreal: McGill-Queens University Press, 309–34.

Chalmers I, Clarke M. (2004) Commentary: The 1944 patulin trial: The first properly controlled multicentre trial conducted under the aegis of the British Medical Research Council. *International Journal of Epidemiology* **32**: 253–60.

Chonde T M. (1980) The role of bacteriological services in the National Tuberculosis and Leprosy Programme in Tanzania. *Bulletin of the International Union Against Tuberculosis and Lung Disease* **64**: 37–9.

Chorine V. (1945) Action de l'amide nicotinique sur les bacilles du genre *Mycobacterium. Comptes Rendus de l'Academie des Sciences* (Paris) **220**: 150–1.

Christie D A, Tansey E M. (eds) (2002) Peptic ulcer: Rise and fall. *Wellcome Witnesses to Twentieth Century Medicine.* Volume 14. London: The Wellcome Trust Centre for the History of Medicine at UCL. Freely available online under publications at www.ucl.ac.uk/histmed

Citron K M. (1972) Tuberculosis – chemotherapy. *British Medical Journal* **i**: 426.

Citron K M. (1988) Control and prevention of tuberculosis in Britain. *British Medical Bulletin* **44**: 704–16.

Citron K M, de Silva D J. (1971) The results of tuberculosis chemotherapy in chest clinic practice. *Tubercle* **52**: 31–6.

Cochrane A L. (1979) 1931–1971: A critical review, with particular reference to the medical profession, in Teeling-Smith G, Wells N. (eds) *Medicines for the Year 2000.* London: Office of Health Economics, 1–11.

Crofton J. (1954) Chemotherapy in pulmonary tuberculosis. *Edinburgh Medical Journal* **61**: 155–69.

Crofton J. (1960) Tuberculosis undefeated. *British Medical Journal* **ii**: 679–87.

Crofton J. (1991) Karel Styblo: A personal tribute. *Bulletin of the International Union Against Tuberculosis and Lung Disease* **66**: 211–3.

Crofton J, Mitchison D A. (1948) Streptomycin resistance in pulmonary tuberculosis. *British Medical Journal* **ii**: 1–18.

Crofton J, Øvreberg K. (1992) Drug resistance and National Tuberculosis Control Programmes (NTP). Unpublished Memorandum in WHO.

Dawson J J Y, Devadatta S, Fox W, Radhakrishna S, Ramakrishnan C V, Somasundaram P R, Stott H, Tripathy S P, Velu S. (1966) A 5-year study of patients with pulmonary tuberculosis in a concurrent comparison of home and sanatorium treatment for one year with isoniazid plus PAS. *Bulletin of the World Health Organization* **34**: 533–51.

Dickinson J M, Mitchison D A. (1968) *In vitro* and *in vivo* studies to assess the suitability of antituberculous drugs for use in intermittent chemotherapy regimens. *Tubercle* **49**: 66–70.

Dickinson J M, Mitchison D A. (1970) Observation *in vitro* on the suitability of pyrazinamide for intermittent chemotherapy of tuberculosis. *Tubercle* **51**: 389–96.

Dickinson J M, Mitchison D A. (1981) Experimental models to explain the high sterilizing activity of rifampin in the chemotherapy of tuberculosis. *American Review of Respiratory Disease* **123**: 367–71.

Dickinson J M, Mitchison D A. (1987) *In vitro* properties of rifapentine (MDL473) relevant to its use in intermittent chemotherapy of tuberculosis. *Tubercle* **68**: 113–8.

Doll R. (1994) Austin Bradford Hill. *Biographical Memoirs of Fellows of the Royal Society* **40**: 128–40.

Dickinson J, Guy A, Mitchison D A. (1992) Bioavailability of rifampicin in experimental murine tuberculosis. *Antimicrobial Agents and Chemotherapy* **36**: 2066–7.

Donald P R, Schoeman J F, Van Zyl L E, De Villiers J N, Pretorius M, Springer P. (1998) Intensive short course chemotherapy in the management of tuberculous meningitis. *International Journal of Tuberculosis and Lung Disease* **2**: 704–11.

Donald P R, Sirgel F A, Venter A, Smit E, Parkin D P, Van de Wal B W, Doré C J, Mitchison D A. (2002) The early bactericidal activity of streptomycin. *International Journal of Tuberculosis and Lung Disease* **6**: 693–8.

Dubovsky H. (1988) The history of para-aminosalicylic acid (PAS), the first tuberculosis anti-microbial agent, and streptomycin (sm): A comparative study. *Adler Museum Bulletin* **14**: 7–11.

East African/[British] Medical Research Council Kenya Tuberculosis Follow-Up. (1970) Tuberculosis in Kenya: A follow-up of a national sampling survey of drug resistance and other factors. *Tubercle* **51**: 1–23.

East African/[British] Medical Research Council. (1960) Comparative trial of isoniazid in combination with thiacetazone or a substituted diphenylthiourea (SU 1906) or PAS in the treatment of acute pulmonary tuberculosis in East Africans. *Tubercle* **41**: 399–423.

East African/[British] Medical Research Council. (1963) Isoniazid with thiacetazone in the treatment of pulmonary tuberculosis in East Africa – second investigation. *Tubercle* **44**: 301–33.

East African/[British] Medical Research Council. (1970) Isoniazid with thiacetazone (thioacetazone) in the treatment of pulmonary tuberculosis in East Africa – fifth investigation. A co-operative study in East African hospitals, clinics and laboratories with the collaboration of the East African and British Medical Research Councils. *Tubercle* **51**: 123–51.

East African/[British] Medical Research Council. (1977) Tuberculosis in Tanzania: A follow-up of a national sampling survey of drug resistance and other factors. *Tubercle* **58**: 55–78.

East African/[British] Medical Research Council. (1978) Controlled clinical trial of five short-course (4-month) chemotherapy regimens in pulmonary tuberculosis. First report of 4th study. *Lancet* **ii**: 334–8.

East African/[British] Medical Research Council. (1979) Tuberculosis in Kenya: Follow-up of the second (1974) national sampling survey and a comparison with the follow-up data from the first (1964) national sampling survey. An East African and British Medical Research Council co-operative investigation. *Tubercle* **60**: 125–49.

Enarson D A. (1995) The International Union Against Tuberculosis and Lung Disease model national tuberculosis programmes. *Tubercle and Lung Disease* **76**: 95–9.

Erdei A (with comment by W E Snell). (1948) Pulmonary tuberculosis treated with para-aminosalicylic acid: Early results in six cases. *Lancet* **i**: 791–3.

Fagerhaugh S, Frankel M. (1970) Behind the scene – it's the skid row hotel manager who sees that Ernie takes his TB drugs. *Bulletin – National Tuberculosis and Respiratory Disease Association* **56**: 12–4.

Ferebee S H. (1970) Controlled chemoprophylaxis trials in tuberculosis. A general review. *Bibliotheca Tuberculosea (Advances in Tuberculosis Research)* **26**: 28–106.

Ferguson G C, Nunn A J, Fox W, Miller A B, Robinson D K, Tall R. (1971) A second international co-operative investigation into thiacetazone side-effects. Rashes on two thiacetazone containing regimens. *Tubercle* 52: 166–81.

Fox H H. (1953) The chemical attack on tuberculosis. *Transactions of the New York Academy of Sciences* **15**: 234–42.

Fox W. (1962a) The chemotherapy and epidemiology of tuberculosis. Some findings of general applicability from the Tuberculosis Chemotherapy Centre, Madras. *Lancet* **ii**: 413–7, 473–8.

Fox W. (1962b) Self-administration of medicaments. A review of published work and a study of the problems, in Proceedings of the XVIth International Tuberculosis Conference, 1961. *Excerpta Medica, International Congress Series* **44**: 1, 307, Amsterdam.

Fox W. (1979) The chemotherapy of pulmonary tuberculosis: A review. *Chest* **76S**: 785–96.

Fox W. (1983a) Compliance of patients and physicians: Experience and lessons from tuberculosis – I. *British Medical Journal* (Clinical Research Edn) **287**: 33–5.

Fox W. (1983b) Compliance of patients and physicians: Experience and lessons from tuberculosis – II. *British Medical Journal (Clinical Research Edn)* **287**: 101–5.

Fox W, Ellard G A, Mitchison D A. (1999) Studies of the treatment of tuberculosis undertaken by the British Medical Research Council Tuberculosis Units, 1946–86, with relevant subsequent publications. *International Journal of Tuberculosis and Lung Disease* **3**: S231–79.

Garrod L P, Lambert H P, O'Grady F. (eds) (1973) Various anti-bacterial antibiotics. *Antibiotic and Chemotherapy.* Chapter 12. 4th edn. Edinburgh: Churchill Livingstone, 220, 446.

Girling D J. (1977) Adverse reactions to rifampicin in antituberculosis regimens. *Journal of Antimicrobial Chemotherapy* **3**: 115–32.

Girling D J. (1978) The hepatic toxicity of antituberculosis regimens containing isoniazid, rifampicin and pyrazinamide. *Tubercle* **59**: 13–32.

Girling D J. (1982) Adverse effects of antituberculosis drugs. *Drugs* **23**: 54–74, also published in *Bulletin of the International Union Against Tuberculosis* 1984; **59**: 152–62.

Girling D J. (1984) The role of pyrazinamide in primary chemotherapy for pulmonary tuberculosis. *Tubercle* **65**: 1–4.

Girling D J. (1989) The chemotherapy of tuberculosis, in Ratledge C, Stanford J, Grange J M. (eds) *The Biology of the Mycobacteria.* Volume 3: *Clinical Aspects of Mycobacterial Disease.* London: Academic Press, 285–323.

Girling D J, Darbyshire J H, Humphries M J, O'Mahoney Sister Gabriel. (1988) Extra-pulmonary tuberculosis. *British Medical Bulletin* **44**: 738–56.

Grosset J. (1971) Georges Canetti (1911–71). *Bulletin of the International Union Against Tuberculosis* **46**: 7–8.

Grosset J. (1978) The sterilizing value of rifampicin and pyrazinamide in experimental short-course chemotherapy. *Tubercle* **59**: 287–97.

Grumbach F, Canetti G, Le Lirzin M. (1969) Rifampicin in daily and intermittent treatment of experimental murine tuberculosis, with emphasis on late results. *Tubercle* **50**: 280–93.

Gyselen A. (1994) Tuberculosis in Belgium: Past, present and future. *Acta Clinica Belgica* **49**: 125–31.

Gyselen A, Simon-Porthier F. (1969) Clinical results in first treatment and retreatment of advanced pulmonary tuberculosis with rifampicin. *Tubercle* **50**: 328–9.

Hakim J G, Ternouth I, Mushangi E, Siziya S, Robertson V, Malin A. (2000) Double blind randomised placebo controlled trial of adjunctive prednisolone in the treatment of effusive tuberculous pericarditis in HIV seropositive patients. *Heart* **84**: 183–8.

Harland R D. (1962) Stevens–Johnson syndrome with unusual skin features occurring in two patients undergoing treatment for pulmonary tuberculosis with thiacetazone. *Tubercle* **43**: 189–91.

Hart P D. (1946) Chemotherapy of tuberculosis – research during the past 100 years. *British Medical Journal* **ii**: 805, 849.

Hart P D. (1999) A change in scientific approach: From alternation to randomized allocation in clinical trials in the 1940s. *British Medical Journal* **319**: 572–3.

Herxheimer A, Zentler-Munro P, Winn D. (1986) *Therapeutic Trials and Society: Making the best use of resources.* A discussion paper. London: Consumers' Association.

Hobby G L. (1982) In memoriam: Walsh McDermott, MD, 1909–81. *American Review of Respiratory Disease* **125**: 141–3.

Hong Kong Antituberculosis Association and Government Tuberculosis Association/[British] Medical Research Council (1968). A controlled comparison of thiacetazone (thio-acetazone) plus isoniazid with PAS plus isoniazid in Hong Kong. *Tubercle* **49**: 243–80.

Hong Kong Chest Service/[British] Medical Research Council. (1977) Controlled trial of 6-month and 9-month regimens of daily and intermittent streptomycin plus isoniazid plus pyrazinamide for pulmonary tuberculosis in Hong Kong. The results up to 30 months. *American Review of Respiratory Disease* **115**: 727–35.

Hong Kong Chest Service/[British] Medical Research Council. (1979) Controlled trial of 6-month and 8-month regimens in the treatment of pulmonary tuberculosis: The results up to 24 months. *Tubercle* **60**: 201–10.

Hong Kong Chest Service/[British] Medical Research Council. (1987) Five-year follow-up of a controlled trial of five 6-month regimens of chemotherapy for pulmonary tuberculosis. *American Review of Respiratory Disease* **136**: 1339–42.

Hong Kong Tuberculosis Treatment Services/[British] Medical Research Council. (1976) Adverse reactions to short-course regimens containing streptomycin, isoniazid, pyrazinamide and rifampicin in Hong Kong. *Tubercle* 57: 81–95.

Hønneland G, Rowe L. (2004) *Health as International Politics. Combating communicable diseases in the Baltic Sea region.* Aldershot: Ashgate Publishing Limited.

Horne N W. (1960) Prednisolone in treatment of pulmonary tuberculosis. A controlled trial. Final report to the Research Committee of the Tuberculosis Society of Scotland. *British Medical Journal* **ii**: 1751–6.

Horne N W, Tulloch W S. (1975) Conservative management of renal tuberculosis. *British Journal of Urology* **47**: 481–7.

Horsfall P A L. (1973) Chemotherapy in the seventies. *Bulletin of the Hong Kong Medical Association* **25**: 23–32.

Humphries M J, Teoh R, Lau J, Gabriel M. (1990) Factors of prognostic significance in Chinese children with tuberculous meningitis. *Tubercle* **71**: 161–8.

Hussain S A, Saksena H C, Kothari R P. (1973) Stevens–Johnson syndrome due to thiacetazone. *Journal of the Indian Medical Association* **60**: 57–9.

International Union Against Tuberculosis. (1964) An international investigation of the efficacy of chemotherapy in previously untreated patients with pulmonary tuberculosis. *Bulletin of the International Union Against Tuberculosis* **34**: 80–191.

International Union Against Tuberculosis and Lung Disease. (1988) Antituberculosis regimens of chemotherapy: Recommendations from the Committee on Treatment of the International Union Against Tuberculosis and Lung Disease. *Bulletin of the International Union Against Tuberculosis and Lung Disease* **63**: 60–4.

Ipuge Y A, Rieder H L, Enarson D A. (1995) Adverse cutaneous reactions to thiacetazone for tuberculosis treatment in Tanzania. *Lancet* **ii**: 657–60.

Iseman M D. (2002) Tuberculosis therapy: Past, present and future. *European Respiratory Journal* **20**: 87S–94S.

Jawahar M S. (2004) Current trends in chemotherapy of tuberculosis. *Indian Journal of Medical Research* **120**: 398–417.

Jindani A. (1976) Short-course (6-month) treatment of pulmonary tuberculosis (Second East African/[British] Medical Research Council Study). *Bulletin of the International Union Against Tuberculosis and Lung Disease* **51**: 53–6.

Jindani A, Aber V R, Edwards E A, Mitchison D A. (1980) The early bactericidal activity of drugs in patients with pulmonary tuberculosis. *American Review of Respiratory Disease* **121**: 939–49.

Jindani A, Doré C J, Mitchison D A. (2003) Bactericidal and sterilizing activities of antituberculosis drugs during the first 14 days. *American Journal of Respiratory and Critical Care Medicine* **167**: 1348–54.

Jindani A, Nunn A J, Enarson D E. (2004) Two 8-month regimens of chemotherapy for treatment of newly diagnosed pulmonary tuberculosis: International multicentred randomized trial. *Lancet* **364**: 1244–51.

Jochem K, Fryatt R J, Harper I, White A, Luitel H, Dahal R. (1997) Tuberculosis control in remote districts of Nepal comparing patient-responsible short-course chemotherapy with long-course treatment. *International Journal of Tuberculosis and Lung Disease* **1**: 502–8.

Joint Tuberculosis Committee of the British Thoracic Society. (1990) Chemotherapy and management of tuberculosis in the United Kingdom: Recommendations of the Joint Tuberculosis Committee of the British Thoracic Society. *Thorax* **45**: 403–40.

Joint Tuberculosis Committee of the British Thoracic Society. (1994) Control and prevention of tuberculosis in the United Kingdom: Code of practice 1994. *Thorax* **49**: 1193–1200.

Joint Tuberculosis Committee of the British Thoracic Society. (1998) Chemotherapy and management of tuberculosis in the United Kingdom: Recommendations 1998. *Thorax* **53**: 536–48.

Joint Tuberculosis Committee of the British Thoracic Society. (2000) Control and prevention of tuberculosis in the United Kingdom: Code of Practice 2000. *Thorax* **55**: 887–901.

Kahana L M. (1996) The problem of drug resistance in tuberculosis. Editorial. *Chest* **110**: 8–9.

Kaplan G, Post F A, Moreira A L, Wainwright H, Kreiswirth B N, Tanverdi M, Mathema B, Ramaswamy S V, Walther G, Steyn L M, Barry C E, Bekker L G. (2003) *Mycobacterium tuberculosis* growth at the cavity surface: A microenvironment with failed immunity. *Infection and Immunity* **71**: 7099–108.

Keers R Y. (1978) *Pulmonary Tuberculosis: A journey down the centuries.* London: Ballière Tindall.

Kent P W, Fox W, Miller A B, Nunn A J, Tall R, Mitchison D A. (1970) The therapy of pulmonary tuberculosis in Kenya: A comparison of the results achieved in controlled clinical trials with those achieved by the routine treatment services. *Tubercle* **51**: 24–38.

Kenyan/[British] Medical Research Council. (1989) Tuberculosis in Kenya 1984: A third national survey and a comparison with earlier surveys in 1964 and 1974. A Kenyan/[British] Medical Research Council Co-operative Investigation. *Tubercle* **70**: 5–20.

Kradolfer F. (1968a) On a new class of bactericidal antibiotics with special reference to rifampicin. [German] *Schweizerische Medizinische Wochenschrift* **98**: 622–7.

Kradolfer F. (1968b) Rifampicin in experimental tuberculosis. [German] *Schweizerische Medizinische Wochenschrift* 98: 1363.

Kritski A L, Rodrigues de Jesus L S, Andrade M K, Werneck-Barroso E, Vieira M A M S, Haffner A, Riley L W. (1997) Editorial. Retreatment tuberculosis cases. Factors associated with drug resistance and adverse outcomes. *Chest* **111**: 1162–7.

Landsborough T A. (1975) *Half a Century of Medical Research.* Volume 1. London: HMSO, 238–9.

Lehmann J. (1946) *Para*-aminosalicylic acid in the treatment of tuberculosis. *Lancet* **i**: 15–16.

MacGregor A R, Stewart S M, Turnbull F W. (1956) The influence of chemotherapy on the bacterial content of tuberculous pulmonary lesions. *Tubercle* **37**: 388–403.

McCune R M, Feldmann F M, Lambert H P, McDermott W. (1966) Microbial persistence. I. The capacity of tubercle bacilli to survive sterilization in mouse tissues. *Journal of Experimental Medicine* **123**: 445–68.

McDermott W. (1952) Isonicotinic acid derivatives in tuberculosis treatment: History of the development of the drugs. *Transactions of the Annual Meeting. National Tuberculosis Association* **48**: 421–4.

McDermott W. (1969) The story of INH. *Journal of Infectious Diseases* **119**: 678–83.

McDermott W. (1970) The John Barnwell lecture: Microbial drug resistance. *American Review of Respiratory Disease* **102**: 857–76.

McDermott W, Ormond L, Muschenheim C, Deuschle K, McCune R M Jr, Tompsett R. (1954) Pyrazinamide–isoniazid in tuberculosis. *American Review of Tuberculosis* **69**: 319–33.

McKenzie D, Malone L, Kuschner S, Oleson J J, Subbarow Y. (1948) The effect of nicotinic acid amide on experimental tuberculosis of white mice. *Journal of Laboratory and Clinical Medicine* **33**: 1249–53.

Medical Research Council, Patulin Clinical Trials Committee. (1944) Clinical trials of patulin in the common cold. *Lancet* **ii**: 373–5.

Medical Research Council. (1948) Streptomycin treatment of pulmonary tuberculosis: A Medical Research Council investigation. *British Medical Journal* **ii**: 769–82.

Medical Research Council. (1955) Various combinations of isoniazid with streptomycin or with PAS in the treatment of pulmonary tuberculosis. *British Medical Journal* **i**: 435–45.

Medical Research Council/Tuberculosis Chemotherapy Trials Committee. (1962) Long-term chemotherapy in the treatment of chronic pulmonary tuberculosis with cavitation. *Tubercle* **43**: 201–67.

Medical Research Council Tuberculosis and Chest Diseases Unit. (1985) Treatment of pulmonary tuberculosis in patients notified in England and Wales in 1978–9; chemotherapy and hospital admission. *Thorax* **40**: 113–20.

Medical Research Council Working Party on Tuberculosis of the Spine. (1976) A five-year assessment of controlled trials of in-patient and out-patient treatment and of plaster-of-Paris jackets for tuberculosis of the spine in children on standard chemotherapy. Studies in Masan and Pusan, Korea. Fifth report. *Journal of Bone and Joint Surgery.* **58-B**: 399–411.

Medical Research Council Working Party on Tuberculosis of the Spine. (1978) Five-year assessments of controlled trials of ambulatory treatment, debridement and anterior spinal fusion in the management of tuberculosis of the spine. Studies in Bulawayo (Rhodesia) and in Hong Kong. Sixth report. *Journal of Bone and Joint Surgery.* **60-B**: 163–77.

Medical Research Council Working Party on Tuberculosis of the Spine. (1999) Five-year assessment of controlled trials of short-course chemotherapy regimens of 6, 9 or 18 months' duration for spinal tuberculosis in patients ambulatory from the start or undergoing radical surgery. Fourteenth report. *International Orthopaedics* **23**: 73–81.

Miller A B, Nunn A J, Robinson D K, Fox W, Somasundaram P R, Tall R. (1972) A second international co-operative investigation into thiacetazone side-effects 2. Frequency and geographical distribution of side-effects. *Bulletin of the World Health Organization* **47**: 211–27.

Mitchison D A. (1973) Plasma concentrations of isoniazid in the treatment of tuberculosis, in Davies D S, Pritchard B N C. (eds) *Biological Effects of Drugs in Relation to Their Plasma Concentrations.* London: Macmillan: 171–82.

Mitchison D A. (1979) Basic mechanisms of chemotherapy. *Chest* **76S**: 771–81S.

Mitchison D A. (1985) The action of antituberculosis drugs in short course chemotherapy. *Tubercle* **66**: 219–25.

Mitchison D A. (1990) Pyrazinamide in the chemoprophylaxis of tuberculosis. *American Review of Respiratory Disease* **142**: 1467.

Mitchison D A. (1998) How drug resistance emerges as a result of poor compliance during short course chemotherapy for tuberculosis. *International Journal of Tuberculosis and Lung Disease* **2**: 10–15.

Mitchison D A. (2004) The search for new sterilizing anti-tuberculosis drugs. *Frontiers in Bioscience* **9**: 1059–72.

Mitchison D A. (2005) The diagnosis and therapy of tuberculosis during the past 100 years. *American Journal of Respiratory and Critical Care Medicine* **171**: 699–706. E-pub 11 February 2005. See www.ajrccm.atsjournals.org/cgi/content/abstract/171/7/699 (visited 6 July 2005).

Mitchison D A, Selkon J B. (1956) The bactericidal activities of antituberculous drugs. *American Review of Respiratory Disease* **74S**: 109–16.

Mitchison D A, Dickinson J M. (1971) Laboratory aspects of intermittent therapy. *Postgraduate Medical Journal* **47**: 737–41.

Mitchison D A, Selkon J B, Weiner A. (1957) A case of pulmonary tuberculosis due to isoniazid-resistant, guinea-pig attenuated, *Mycobacterium tuberculosis. Tubercle* **38**: 382–6.

Mitchison D A, Ellard G A, Grosset J. (1988) New antibacterial drugs for the treatment of mycobacterial disease in man. *British Medical Bulletin* **44**: 757–74.

Monie R D, Hunter A M, Rocchiccioli K, White J, Campbell I A, Kilpatrick G S. (1982) Survey of pulmonary tuberculosis in south and west Wales (1976–8). *British Medical Journal* **284**: 571–3.

Mudie I S, Horne N W, Crofton J W. (1954) Isoniazid and weight gain. *British Medical Journal* **i**: 1304–5.

Murray C J, Styblo K, Rouillon A. (1990) Tuberculosis in developing countries: Burden, intervention and cost. *Bulletin of the International Union Against Tuberculosis and Lung Disease* **65**: 6–24.

Murray C J, DeJonghe E, Chum H J, Nyangulu D S, Salomao A, Styblo K. (1991) Cost effectiveness of chemotherapy for pulmonary tuberculosis in three sub-Saharan African countries. *Lancet* **338**: 1305–8.

Ntsekhe M, Wiysonge C, Volmink J A, Commerford P J, Mayosi B M. (2003) Adjuvant corticosteroids for tuberculous pericarditis: Promising, but not proven. *Quarterly Journal of Medicine* **96**: 593–9.

Nuermberger E L, Yoshimatsu T, Tyagi S, O'Brien R J, Vernon A N, Chaisson R E, Bishai W R, Grosset J H. (2004a) Moxifloxacin-containing regimen greatly reduces time to culture conversion in murine tuberculosis. *American Journal of Respiratory and Critical Care Medicine* **169**: 421–6.

Nuermberger E L, Yoshimatsu T, Tyagi S, Williams K, Rosenthal I, O'Brien R J, Vernon A A, Chaisson R E, Bishai W R, Grosset J H. (2004b) Moxifloxacin-containing regimens of reduced duration produce a stable cure in murine tuberculosis. *American Journal of Respiratory and Critical Care Medicine* **170**: 1131–4.

O'Brien R J. (1989) Present chemotherapy of tuberculosis. *Seminars in Respiratory Infections* **4**: 216–24.

O'Mahoney G, Wing-kar C. (1973) Relationship between rifampicin-dependent antibody scores, serum rifampicin concentrations and symptoms in patients with adverse reactions to intermittent rifampicin treatment. *Clinical Allergy* **3**: 353–62.

Ormerod L P. (2001) The clinical management of the drug-resistant patient. *Annals of the New York Academy of Sciences* **953**: 185–91.

Ormerod L P, Prescott R T. (2003) The management of pulmonary and lymph node tuberculosis notified in England and Wales in 1998. *Clinical Medicine* **3**: 57–61.

Pomerantz M, Brown J M. (1997) Surgery in the treatment of multidrug-resistant tuberculosis. *Clinics in Chest Medicine* **18**: 123–30.

Ramakrishnan C V, Rajendran K, Mohan K, Fox W, Radhakrishna S. (1966) The diet, physical activity and accommodation of patients with quiescent pulmonary tuberculosis in a poor South Indian community. *Bulletin of the World Health Organization* **34**: 553–71.

Reynolds L A, Tansey E M. (eds) (2001) Childhood asthma and beyond. *Wellcome Witnesses to Twentieth Century Medicine.* Volume 11. London: The Wellcome Trust Centre for the History of Medicine at UCL. Freely available online under publications at www.ucl.ac.uk/histmed

Riska N. (1976) Hepatitis cases in isoniazid treated groups and in a control group. *Bulletin of the International Union Against Tuberculosis* **51**: 203–8.

Ross J D, Horne N W, Grant I W B, Crofton J W. (1958) Hospital treatment of pulmonary tuberculosis: a follow-up study of patients admitted to Edinburgh hospitals in 1953. *British Medical Journal* **i**: 237–42.

Sackett D L, Snow J C. (1979). The magnitude of compliance and non-compliance, in Haynes R B, Taylor D W, Sackett D L. (eds) *Compliance in Health Care.* Baltimore: Johns Hopkins University Press, 11–22.

Saerens E J. (1972) Rifampicin: A first line tuberculostatic drug. A critical review and appraisal. *Acta Tuberculosea et Pneumologica Belgica* **63**: 516–28.

Schatz A, Bugie E, Waksman S A. (1944) Streptomycin, a substance exhibiting antibiotic activity against gram-positive and gram-negative bacteria. *Proceedings of the Society for Experimental Biology and Medicine* **55**: 66–9.

Schurr E, Buschman E, Malo D, Gros P, Skamene E. (1990) Immunogenetics of mycobacterial infections: Mouse–human homologies. *Journal of Infectious Diseases* **161**: 634–9.

Scottish Thoracic Society. (1963) A controlled trial of chemotherapy in pulmonary tuberculosis of doubtful activity, 5-year follow-up. *Tubercle* **44**: 39–46.

Sensi P. (1983) History of the development of rifampin. *Reviews of Infectious Diseases* **5**: S402–6.

Sirgel F A, Fourie P B, Donald P R, Padayatchi N, Rustomjee R, Levin J, Roscigno G, Norman J, McIlleron H, Mitchison D A. (2005) The early bactericidal activities of rifampin and rifapentine in pulmonary tuberculosis. *American Journal of Respiratory and Critical Care Medicine* (E-pub ahead of print 1 April 2005). See www.ajrccm.atsjournals.org/cgi/content/abstract/172/1/128 (visited 6 July 2005).

Snell W E. (1978) *The British Thoracic Association: The first fifty years.* London: British Thoracic Association.

Snider D E Jr, Zierski M, Graczyk J, Bek E, Farer L S. (1986) Short-course tuberculosis chemotherapy studies conducted in Poland during the past decade. *European Journal of Respiratory Diseases* **68**: 12–18.

Somner A R. (1975) Proceedings: Short course chemotherapy in pulmonary tuberculosis: A controlled trial by the British Thoracic and Tuberculosis Association. (A report from one of the three clinical co-ordinators.) *Tubercle* **56**: 165.

Spinaci S. (1990) Tuberculosis in the 90s – a world challenge in the WHO perspective with special reference to the Eastern IUATLD region, in *Short-course Chemotherapy for National Tuberculosis Control Programmes in Developing Countries.* Proceeding of a symposium held in Beijing Republic of China. Oxford: Medical Publishing Foundation, 7–14.

Strang J I G, Gibson D G, Nunn A J, Kakaza H H S, Girling D J, Fox W. (1987) Controlled trial of prednisolone as adjuvant in treatment of tuberculous constrictive pericarditis in Transkei. *Lancet* **ii**: 1418–22.

Strang J I G, Kakaza H H S, Gibson D G, Allen B W, Mitchison D A, Evans D J, Girling D J, Nunn A J, Fox W. (1988) Controlled clinical trial of complete open surgical drainage and of prednisolone in treatment of tuberculous pericardial effusion in Transkei. *Lancet* **ii**: 759–64.

Strang J I G, Nunn A J, Johnson D A, Casbard A, Gibson D G, Girling D J. (2004) Management of tuberculous constrictive pericarditis and tuberculous pericardial effusion in Transkei: Results at ten years follow-up. *Quarterly Journal of Medicine* **97**: 525–35.

Sutherland I. (1998) Medical Research Council Streptomycin Trial, in Armitage P, Colton T. (eds) *Encyclopaedia of Biostatistics*. Chichester: John Wiley and Sons **3**: 2554–62.

Tansey E M. (2004) Philip Montagu D'Arcy Hart. The James Lind Library (www.jameslindlibrary.org) visited 1 June 2005.

Tansey E M, Reynolds L A. (2000) Post penicillin antibiotics: From acceptance to resistance? *Wellcome Witnesses to Twentieth Century Medicine*. Volume 6. London: The Wellcome Trust Centre for the History of Medicine at UCL. Freely available online under publications at www.ucl.ac.uk/histmed

Tanzanian/[British] Medical Research Council. (1985) Tuberculosis in Tanzania – a national survey of newly notified cases. Tanzanian/British Medical Research Council Collaborative Study. *Tubercle* **66**: 161–78.

Thwaites G E, Nguyen D B, Nguyen H D, Hoang T Q, Do T T, Nguyen T C, Nguyen Q H, Nguyen T T, Nguyen N H, Nguyen T N, Nguyen N L, Nguyen H D, Vu N T, Cao H H, Tran T H, Pham P M, Nguyen T D, Stepniewska K, White N J, Tran T H, Farrar J J. (2004) Dexamethasone for the treatment of tuberculous meningitis in adolescents and adults. *New England Journal of Medicine* **351**: 1741–51.

Tuberculosis Chemotherapy Centre, Madras. (1959) A concurrent comparison of home and sanatorium treatment of pulmonary tuberculosis in South India. *Bulletin of the World Health Organization* **21**: 51–144.

Tuberculosis Chemotherapy Centre, Madras. (1960) A concurrent comparison of isoniazid plus PAS with three regimens of isoniazid alone in the domiciliary treatment of pulmonary tuberculosis in South India. *Bulletin of the World Health Organization* **23**: 535–85.

Tuberculosis Chemotherapy Centre, Madras. (1963a) The prevention and treatment of isoniazid toxicity in the therapy of pulmonary tuberculosis 1. An assessment of two vitamin B preparations and glutamic acid. *Bulletin of the World Health Organization* **28**: 455–75.

Tuberculosis Chemotherapy Centre, Madras. (1963b) The prevention and treatment of isoniazid toxicity in the therapy of pulmonary tuberculosis 2. An assessment of the prophylactic effect of pyridoxine in low dosage. *Bulletin of the World Health Organization* **29**: 457–81.

Tuberculosis Chemotherapy Trials Committee. (1952) The treatment of pulmonary tuberculosis with isoniazid. *British Medical Journal* **ii**: 735–46.

Tuberculosis Research Centre, Madras. (1983) Study of chemotherapy regimens of 5 and 7 months' duration and the role of corticosteroids in the treatment of sputum-positive patients with pulmonary tuberculosis in South India. *Tubercle* **64**: 73–91.

Tuberculosis Society of Scotland. (1960) The treatment of pulmonary tuberculosis at work: A controlled trial. *Tubercle* **41**: 161–70.

Tucker W B. (1955) Comparative efficacy of the streptomycin and para-aminosalicylic acid regimens of prolonged duration in patients with previously untreated pulmonary tuberculosis. *American Review of Tuberculosis* **72**: 733–55.

Voskuil M I, Schnappinger D, Visconti K C, Harrell M I, Dolganov G M, Sherman D R, Schoolnik G K. (2003) Inhibition of respiration by nitric oxide induces a *Mycobacterium tuberculosis* dormancy program. *Journal of Experimental Medicine* **198**: 705–13.

Waksman S A, Woodruff H B. (1940) The soil as a source of microorganisms antagonistic to disease producing bacteria. *Journal of Bacteriology* **40**: 581–600.

Wallace A T, Stewart S M, Turnbull F A, Crofton J W. (1954) Isoniazid resistance in patients with pulmonary tuberculosis treated on isoniazid alone. *Tubercle* **35**: 164–70.

Wehrli W, Staehelin M. (1969) The rifamycins – relation of chemical structure and action on RNA polymerase. *Biochimica et Biophysica Acta* **182**: 24–9.

Wilkinson D, Moore D A. (1996) HIV-related tuberculosis in South Africa – clinical features and outcome. *South African Medical Journal* **86**: 64–7.

Wilkinson L. (1997) Sir Austin Bradford Hill: Medical statistics and the quantitative approach to prevention of disease. *Addiction* **92**: 657–66.

World Health Organization. (1994) WHO Tuberculosis Programme: Framework for effective tuberculosis control. *WHO/TB* **94**: 179.

World Health Organization. (1999) What is DOTS? A guide to understanding the WHO-recommended TB control strategy known as DOTS. *WHO/CDS/CPC/TB/* **99**: 270. Geneva, Switzerland: World Health Organization; see also www.who.int/gtb/dots (visited 28 June 2005).

Worlledge S. (1973a) The detection of rifampicin-dependent antibodies. *Scandinavian Journal of Respiratory Disease* **84** (supplement): 60–63.

Worlledge S. (1973b) Correlation between the presence of rifampicin-dependent antibodies and the clinical data. *Scandinavian Journal of Respiratory Disease* **84** (supplement): 125–8.

Yoshioka A. (1998) Use of randomisation in the Medical Research Council's clinical trial of streptomycin in pulmonary tuberculosis in the 1940s. *British Medical Journal* **ii**: 1220–3.

Zhang Y, Mitchison D. (2003) The curious characteristics of pyrazinamide: A review. *International Journal of Tuberculosis and Lung Disease* 7: 6–21.

Biographical notes*

Dr Joseph Angel
(b. 1923) was coordinator of the British Thoracic Association's trial of short-course chemotherapy in tuberculosis from 1972 to 1984. He had previously conducted clinical trials in tuberculosis at the State University of New York (1957–8) and as Medical Officer at the joint WHO/MRC Tuberculosis Chemotherapy Centre in Madras, South India, under the direction or Dr Wallace Fox (1959–60). From 1964 to 1989 he was Consultant Physician to Watford General and Harefield Hospitals (Middlesex).

Sir Christopher Booth
Kt FRCP (b. 1924) trained as a gastroenterologist and was the first Convenor of the Wellcome Trust's History of Twentieth Century Medicine Group, from 1990 to 1996, and Harveian Librarian at the Royal College of Physicians from 1989 to 1997. He was Professor of Medicine at the Royal Postgraduate Medical School, Hammersmith Hospital, London, from 1966 to 1977 and Director of the Medical Research Council's Clinical Research Centre, Northwick Park Hospital, Harrow, from 1978 to 1988.

Sir Austin Bradford Hill
Kt CBE FRS (1897–1991) was Professor of Medical Statistics at the London School of Hygiene and Tropical Medicine from 1945 until 1961. See Doll (1994).

Dr Ian Campbell
FRCP (b. 1944), a chest physician in Cardiff, was one of the coordinators of the first British trial of short-course chemotherapy and coordinated the first randomized trial of chemotherapy for lymph node tuberculosis. He has retained his interest in tuberculosis, has been Honorary Secretary, and currently is Chairman of the Joint Tuberculosis Committee of the British Thoracic Society. He was President of the Society in 2003.

Sir Iain Chalmers
Kt FRCPE FFPHM FMedSci (b. 1943) is editor of the James Lind Library (www.jameslindlibrary.org), a web-based resource containing material about the history of the development of methods to test the effects of medical treatments. He was Director of the UK Cochrane Centre, Oxford, between 1992 and

*Contributors are asked to supply details; other entries are compiled from conventional biographical sources.

2002, and Director of the National Perinatal Epidemiology Unit, Oxford, from 1978 to 1992.

Dr Kenneth Citron
FRCP (b. 1925) was Consultant Physician in Respiratory Medicine at the Royal Brompton Hospital London, from 1959 to 1990, President of the British Thoracic Society (1986–8) and Chairman of its Tuberculosis Clinical Trials Committee and Joint Tuberculosis Committee (1971–88). He was also Consultant Adviser on Tuberculosis to the Department of Health (1976–87).

Sir John Crofton
Kt FRCP (b. 1912) was Professor of Respiratory Diseases and Tuberculosis at the University of Edinburgh from 1952 until his retirement in 1977. From 1947 to 1950, he worked part-time at the MRC Tuberculosis Unit at the Brompton Hospital, London, and as Lecturer, later Senior Lecturer, at the Royal Postgraduate Medical School, Hammersmith Hospital, London, from 1947 to 1951. He was a member of the MRC Tuberculosis Chemotherapy Trials Committee from 1952 to 1963.

Professor Janet Darbyshire
OBE FRCP FMedSci (b. 1947) joined the MRC Tuberculosis and Chest Diseases Unit in 1974, where she coordinated clinical trials and epidemiological studies in Africa and the UK until 1989. Subsequently she has been responsible for a programme of clinical trials in HIV infection and now, as Director of the MRC Clinical Trials Unit, also in cancer and other disease areas.

Dr Peter Davies
(b. 1949) has been Consultant Chest Physician and Director of the Tuberculosis Research and Resource Unit, Cardiothoracic Centre and Aintree University Hospital, Liverpool, since 1988, and Honorary Professor, University of Liverpool, since May 2004. He completed his DM thesis on the epidemiology of tuberculosis in England and Wales while working as a Clinical Scientific Officer at the MRC Tuberculosis and CDU (1978–80). He is editor of *Clinical Tuberculosis*, 3rd edn. London: Hodder Arnold, 2003.

Mrs Caroline Doré
(b. 1949) graduated in statistics from University College London. She was a consultant statistician for the MRC Environmental Physiology Research Unit, MRC Clinical Research Centre, Royal Postgraduate Medical School, London, and became Head of the Statistical Consultancy Service for Imperial College School of

Medicine. Since 2001 she has been the Senior Statistician for the Arthritis Research Campaign Clinical Trials Collaboration, based at the MRC Clinical Trials Unit.

Dr Freda Festenstein
(b. 1927) was assistant chest physician at the London Chest Hospital from 1963 to 1989 and full-time Consultant Physician with a special interest in tuberculosis, its epidemiology and control, and honorary senior lecturer in the National Heart and Lung Institute, London Chest Hospital from 1989 to 1992. Following her retirement in September 1992 she became honorary senior lecturer attached to the Department of Microbiology with Dr John Grange in 1993, in the Royal Brompton National Heart and Lung Institute. She has since maintained an active interest in the International Union Against Tuberculosis and Lung Disease.

Professor Wallace Fox
CMG FRCP FFCM (b. 1920) was Professor of Community Therapeutics at the Brompton Hospital, London, from 1979 to 1986, and Director of the MRC Tuberculosis and Chest Diseases Unit from 1965 to 1986. He has been WHO Consultant from 1961 and was seconded to WHO to establish and direct the Tuberculosis Chemotherapy Centre, Madras, from 1956 to 1961 (see Appendix 1).

Dr David Girling
FRCP (b. 1937), following appointments in chest medicine and neonatal research, joined the MRC Tuberculosis and Chest Diseases Unit in 1971 and coordinated tuberculosis trials in Hong Kong, Singapore, Czechoslovakia and Transkei. He served on the Committee on Treatment of the International Union Against Tuberculosis and Lung Disease, drafting this committee's recommendations on antituberculosis chemotherapy. He took a particular interest in adverse effects of antituberculosis drugs. At the MRC Clinical Trials Unit, he coordinated the programmes of lung cancer and upper gastrointestinal tract cancer trials and currently chairs a Data Monitoring and Ethics Committee for the Christie Hospital, Manchester.

Professor Alan Glynn
FRCP FRCPath (b. 1923) qualified at University College Hospital, London. He trained in clinical medicine but after two years as a senior registrar at St Mary's Hospital, London, he converted to bacteriology becoming Professor

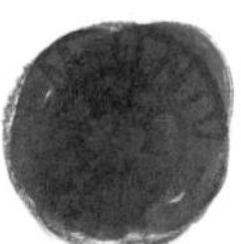

there in 1971 and Head of the Department of Bacteriology in 1974. In 1980 he became Director of the Central Public Health Laboratory at Colindale, London until his retirement in 1988.

Professor John Grange
(b. 1943) was Reader in Clinical Microbiology at the National Heart and Lung Institute, Imperial College, London, from 1976 to 2000, and is currently a Visiting Professor at the Centre for Infectious Diseases and International Health, Royal Free and University College Medical School, London.

Dr Jacques Grosset
(b. 1929) was Professor of Bacteriology, Virology, and Hygiene, at the Faculty of Medicine Pitié-Salpêtrière, Paris, France (1970–99), Emeritus Professor of Bacteriology, Virology and Hygiene (1999–present) and has been Visiting Professor, Center for Tuberculosis Research, Johns Hopkins School of Medicine, Maryland, since 2001.

Dr Philip D'Arcy Hart
CBE FRCP Hon FMedSci (b. 1900) trained in medicine at University College London, where he became a Consultant Physician. He was Director of the MRC Tuberculosis Research Unit from 1948 until his retirement in 1965. See Tansey (2004).

Dr Elizabeth Hills
MBE FRCP (b. 1935) was Consultant Physician in Aylesbury (1969–79) and has worked in the Mukeza District Designated Hospital, Tanzania, from 1980–91, and 1994–2001, being Medical Superintendent there from 1982. From 1970 to 1979 she was a member of the BTA/BTS Research Committee.

Dr Peter Anthony (Tony) Jenkins
(b. 1936) graduated from University College Cardiff and from 1960–5 was Assistant Lecturer, MRC Clinical Immunology Research Group, Institute of Diseases of the Chest, Brompton Hospital, London. He obtained his PhD from the University of London in 1964 for 'Immunological Studies in Farmer's Lung'. From 1965 to 1977 he was Principal Scientific Officer, at the Tuberculosis Reference Laboratory (PHLS), Cardiff, and from 1977 to 1995, Head of the Mycobacterium Reference Unit (PHLS), Cardiff.

Dr Amina Jindani
FRCP (b. 1936) has held various posts as coordinator of clinical trials at the MRC's Tuberculosis and Chest Diseases Unit, London, the East African Tuberculosis Investigation Centre (1967–77), at the Department of Preventive Medicine and Biostatistics of the University of Toronto (1977–80)

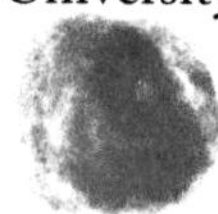

and at the International Union Against Tuberculosis and Lung Disease, Paris (1997–2004). She is currently Honorary Senior Lecturer in the Department of Cellular and Molecular Medicine at St George's Hospital Medical School, London, where she is involved in establishing international multicentre clinical trials in tuberculosis.

Dr Pierce Kent
OBE (b. 1914) was Director of the East Africa Tuberculosis Investigations Centre, Nairobi. This was an East African Community Research Centre that carried out prevalence surveys as well as clinical trials in tuberculosis in Kenya, Uganda and Tanzania.

Dr Adrian Martineau
(b. 1971) is a clinical research fellow at the Wellcome Centre for Research in Clinical Tropical Medicine, Imperial College, London.

Dr Walsh McDermott
(1909–81) was Professor of Public Health and Medicine at the Cornell University Medical College, New York, and Chairman of the Department of Public Health (1955–72). He helped develop antimicrobial drugs for the treatment of tuberculosis and in 1955 received the Albert Lasker Award for development of the antituberculosis drug isoniazid. See Hobby (1982); *New York Times* 19 October, 1981.

Dr Jeanette Meadway
(b. 1947) was registrar and senior registrar in respiratory medicine, Aylesbury and St Mary's Hospital, London, between 1972 and 1980. In 1981 she became consultant physician in Newham, London. From 1985 she worked increasingly with tuberculosis and HIV, becoming lead clinician in infection and immunity in 1996. Since 1997 she has been consultant physician at Mildmay Mission Hospital, London, an HIV rehabilitation and palliative care unit.

Professor Denis (Denny) Mitchison
CMG FRCP FRCPath (b. 1919) was Professor of Bacteriology at the Royal Postgraduate Medical School, Hammersmith Hospital, London, from 1971 until his retirement in 1985 (Emeritus Professor until 1993) and Emeritus Professor at St George's Hospital Medical School, London, since 1993. He was Director of the MRC's Unit for Laboratory Studies of Tuberculosis from 1956 until 1984, and collaborated with the MRC Tuberculosis Research Unit (from 1968 the Tuberculosis and Chest Diseases Unit) in developing effective chemotherapy for

tuberculosis and research laboratories in East Africa, Madras, Hong Kong, Singapore and Prague. He performed the laboratory tests for the 1948 Tuberculosis Chemotherapy Committee Report and was a member of the 1952 Committee.

Dr John Moore-Gillon

FRCP (b. 1953) is a Consultant Physician at St Bartholomew's and The Royal London Hospitals, London. He is lead clinician for tuberculosis for the London Borough of Tower Hamlets, formerly Honorary Secretary and now Chairman of the Joint Tuberculosis Committee, and formerly Chairman and now President of the British Lung Foundation.

Professor Andrew Nunn

(b. 1943) was the senior statistician in the MRC Tuberculosis and Chest Diseases Unit, from 1972 to 1986. Following the closure of the Unit he worked in Uganda for six years on the MRC AIDS Programme; in 1998 he became Head of the Division Without Portfolio, MRC Clinical Trials Unit, with responsibility for developing trials in neglected areas.

Professor Lawrence (Peter) Ormerod

FRCP (b. 1950) was appointed Chest Physician in Blackburn, a high Tuberculosis District in 1980. He was awarded his MD (1986) and DSc (2000) for tuberculosis clinical and operational research. He has been a member of the Joint Tuberculosis Committee since 1987 (Chair from 1995 to 2000) and a Consultant Adviser on Tuberculosis to the Department of Health, 1997–2003. He has written widely on tuberculosis with over 70 peer-reviewed papers.

Dr Knut Øvreberg

(b. 1928) was Head of the Troms County Chest Clinic in Harstad, Norway, (1968–93), when he retired. He worked with Dr Karel Styblo in Paris and in Mozambique from 1982 until 1992. He has been a member of the Tuberculosis Committee of the Britain–Nepal Medical Trust and during the first years with Dr Wallace Fox and Sir John Crofton.

Dr Geoff Scott

(b. 1948) has been Consultant Clinical Microbiologist at University College London Hospitals since 1984. He manages patients with tuberculosis.

Dr Joe Selkon
FRCPath (b. 1928) was a microbiologist on the staff of the Medical Research Council Unit for research into drug sensitivity in tuberculosis, and subsequently in charge of the microbiology laboratory of the World Health Organization, Tuberculosis Chemotherapy Centre, Madras, India. He was Consultant Microbiologist and Director of the Oxford Regional Public Health Laboratory; Honorary Clinical Lecturer, University of Oxford; Chairman of the Research Committee of the British Tuberculosis and Thoracic Association from 1973 to 1976; and President of the British Thoracic Society from 1988 to 1993. He was awarded the Dorothy Temple Cross Fellowship for research in tuberculosis in 1958.

Dr Alan Somner
FRCPEd (b. 1923) qualified in Edinburgh in 1946, trained at the Edinburgh Respiratory Diseases Unit and was Consultant Physician in Respiratory Medicine, North Tyneside, from 1960 to 1984. He coordinated several national clinical trials in Britain on tuberculosis among immigrants and chemotherapy for tuberculosis on behalf of the British Thoracic Association, and was their President from 1981 to 1982.

Dr Bertie Squire
FRCP (b. 1960) trained in infectious diseases and tropical medicine. He was Head of the Medical Department, Kanuzu Central Hospital, Lilongwe, Malawi, between 1992 and 1995. Since 1995 he has been Senior Lecturer in Clinical Tropical Medicine at the Liverpool School of Tropical Medicine. He manages a research programme on tuberculosis, which is funded by the UK's Department for International Development.

Dr Karel Styblo
(1922–98) was scientific director of the International Union Against Tuberculosis and Lung Disease (IUATLD) in Paris (1979–91) and developed the tuberculosis control strategy known as DOTS. See Crofton (1991).

Glossary

Chemoprophylaxis
The use of a chemotherapeutic agent as a means of preventing development of a specific disease.

Culture
A laboratory test in which tubercle bacilli present in biological specimens such as sputum are grown on a suitable culture medium. The susceptibility of the cultured bacilli to various antituberculosis drugs can then be assessed. Culture incubation can take four or more weeks.

Extrapulmonary tuberculosis
Tuberculous disease in any part of the body other than the lungs (for example, the kidney or lymph nodes).

Fully supervised chemotherapy
Every single dose of a regimen is given under the direct supervision of tuberculosis service staff, orally administered drugs being seen to be swallowed and the patient's mouth shown to be empty afterwards.

Mycobacterium
A genus of bacteria of the family Mycobacteriaceae, order Actinomycetales, occurring as Gram-positive, aerobic and mostly slow-growing. The most characteristic feature of cultures of mycobacteria is that they are acid fast.

Pro-drug
A drug that enters cells more easily and only there gets converted to the wanted active molecule.

Stevens–Johnson syndrome *(Erythema multiforme)*
Severe red and blistering eruptions of skin and mucous membranes, accompanied by high fever. An important and often fatal reaction, notably in patients with HIV/TB, to chemotherapy drugs, particularly thiacetazone.

Streptomyces
A genus of fungus-like bacteria of the family Streptomycetaceae, order Actinomycetales.

Tuberculosis (TB)
A disease caused by the bacterium *Mycobacterium tuberculosis* (tubercle bacillus) which most commonly affects the lungs (pulmonary tuberculosis) but can also affect the central nervous system (meninges; brain and spinal cord), lymphatic system, genitourinary system, bones, joints and other organs/tissues. Miliary tuberculosis is widespread dissemination of the bacilli in the body.

Abbreviations

ACE = Angiotensin-converting enzyme
ACTH = Adrenocorticotrophic hormone
ATS = American Thoracic Society
BTA = British Thoracic Association
BTS = British Thoracic Society
BTTA = British Thoracic and Tuberculosis Association
DOT = Directly observed therapy
DOTS = Directly observed therapy, short-course strategy
E = Ethambutol
EHR = Ethambutol, isoniazid and rifampicin
ERS = European Respiratory Society
FDC = Fixed-dose combination
H = Isoniazid
HPA = Health Protection Agency
HRE = Isoniazid, rifampicin and ethambutol
HRZ = Isoniazid, rifampicin and pyrazinamide
HRZE = Isoniazid, rifampicin, pyrazinamide and ethambutol
ICMR = Indian Council of Medical Research
INAH = Isoniazid
IRS = Immune reconstitution syndrome
IUATLD = International Union Against Tuberculosis and Lung Disease
MDR = Multidrug-resistant
MRC = Medical Research Council
NICE = National Institute for Clinical Excellence
PAS = Para-aminosalicylic acid
PHLS = Public Health Laboratory Service
PHS = Public Health Service
R = Rifampicin
3RH = Three months of daily rifampicin and isoniazid
RZ = Rifampicin and pyrazinamide
S = Streptomycin
TB = Tuberculosis
TCDU = Tuberculosis and Chest Diseases Unit
WHO = World Health Organization
Z = Pyrazinamide

Index: Subject

Index: Names

Biographical notes appear in bold

Key to cover photographs

Front cover, top to bottom

Dr David Girling, Chair

Professor Denny Mitchison

Sir John Crofton

Dr Joseph Angel

Back cover, top to bottom

Dr Kenneth Citron

Dr Ian Campbell, Professor Peter Ormerod

Professor Andrew Nunn

Dr Joseph Angel, Professor Janet Darbyshire, Professor Alan Glynn

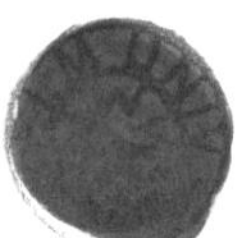

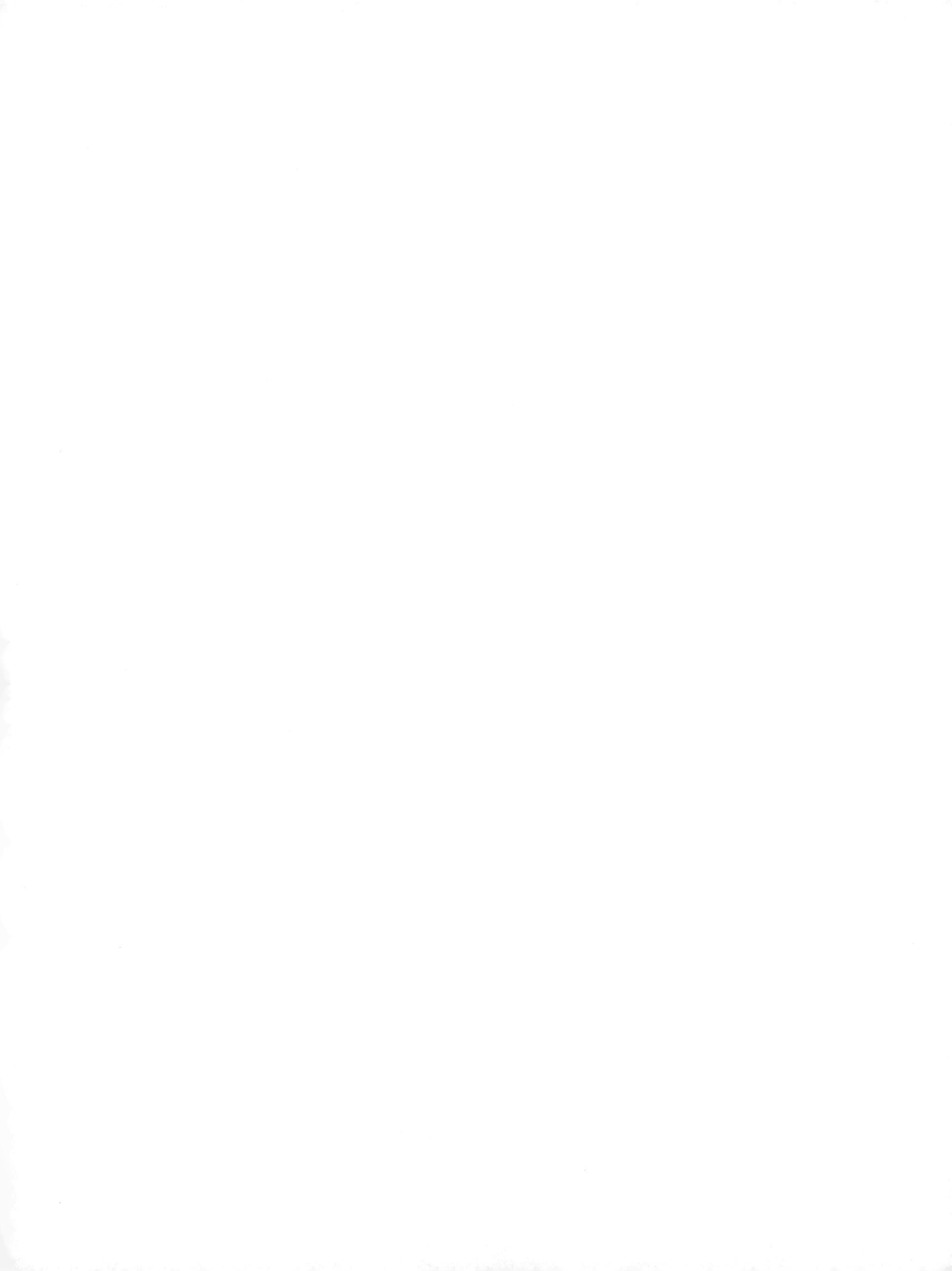

CPSIA information can be obtained at www.ICGtesting.com
Printed in the USA
LVOW051503290512

283769LV00007B/4/A